The Natural Way
for Dogs & Cats

MIDI FAIRGRIEVE

The Natural Way for Dogs & Cats

Natural treatments, remedies
and diet for your pet

ILLUSTRATED BY JANE NORMAN

SAFFRON WALDEN
THE C.W. DANIEL COMPANY LIMITED

First published in Great Britain by
Mainstream Publishing, Edinburgh

This totally revised and expanded edition published in 2001 by
The C.W. Daniel Company Limited,
1 Church Path, Saffron Walden, Essex, CB10 1JP,
United Kingdom

© Midi Fairgrieve 1998 & 2001

ISBN 0 85207 344 5 3695 5457 3108

Produced in association with
Book Production Consultants plc, 25–27 High Street,
Chesterton, Cambridge, CB4 1ND
Typeset by Cambridge Photosetting Services
Printed and bound by Biddles, Guildford, England

Contents

	Acknowledgements	vii
	Foreword	ix
Chapter 1	Introduction	1
Chapter 2	Ten tips to keep your pet happy and healthy	5
Chapter 3	It's simple, isn't it?	7
Chapter 4	A healthy diet	9
Chapter 5	Food supplements	28
Chapter 6	Vaccinations	41
Chapter 7	Acupuncture	45
Chapter 8	Aromatherapy	54
Chapter 9	Biochemical tissue salts	65
Chapter 10	Chiropractic	70
Chapter 11	Flower essences	77
Chapter 12	Healing	91
Chapter 13	Herbal medicine	101
Chapter 14	Homoeopathy	117

Chapter 15	T-touch massage	130
Chapter 16	Natural remedies for first-aid use	136
Chapter 17	Specific ailments and treatments	146
	Behavioural problems	149
	Cancer	155
	Cardiovascular system	156
	Digestive problems	159
	Ear problems	176
	Eye problems	178
	Immune system and infectious diseases	180
	Kidney and urinary problems	182
	Muscle and joint problems	186
	Operations	193
	Parasites	194
	Pregnancy and associated problems	200
	Respiratory system	204
	Skin and coat	207
	Spaying and neutering	214
	General resources	216
	Bibliography	218
	At-a-glance guide to the Bach Flower Remedies	220
	Index	221

Acknowledgements

I would like to thank the following people for helping me with my research for this book and for giving their time and expertise freely and willingly: the Hon. Richard Arthur (McTimoney chiropractic), Christy Casley (healing), Keren Brynes (herbal medicine), Mary Boughton (herbal medicine), Sarah Fisher (aromatherapy and T-touch), Helen Gould (acupuncture), Dana Green (McTimoney chiropractic), Clare Harvey (flower essences), Daniel M. Iannarelli (osteopathy), Alasdair MacFarlane Govan (acupuncture), Christine Newman (Bach flower remedies), John A. Rohrbach (herbal medicine), June Third-Carter (homoeopathy), and The Self-Realization Meditation Healing Centre, Somerset (healing).

I would also like to thank the following friends and family members for their unflagging help and support throughout the writing of this book: Pat Agnew, Laura Borkovy, Alison De Marco, Rosie Filipiak and Steve Godfrey.

Foreword

I first began working with animals 10 years ago as a spiritual healer and was constantly amazed by their positive response to this gentle, yet powerful natural therapy. At the same time I was practising nutritional medicine with people. Although I also gave healing to people, I didn't practise nutritional medicine on animals. That is, until I got my dog, Basil. After a few months of feeding him what I considered a good-quality, 'complete' dried food every day, I began to think – why am I doing this when I know the much greater health benefits of a fresh, natural, preservative-free diet, such as I was eating myself and recommending to all of my human patients? That thought was the start of an exploration into canine and feline nutrition, followed by research into the use of many other natural treatments and remedies that work wonderfully with animals. Nowadays, I combine all my knowledge as a healer, counsellor and practitioner of nutritional medicine to treat both animals and people.

This book is to help you on your way to making healthier choices for your pet, practising preventative measures and ensuring their diet, the cornerstone of good health, is as good as it can be. When your pet's health is built upon a solid foundation of good diet, you will rarely need to take them to a vet or complementary health practitioner.

CHAPTER ONE

Introduction

Nature has always held a cure for disease and it is only natural that we are returning to her for the answers, both for ourselves and for our animals. It is easy to forget that, before modern medicine, people and animals looked to nature for a cure. It is not surprising then that as more and more people are choosing natural treatments and remedies for themselves they are also seeking them for their pets.

It is also becoming easier to find someone who will treat your pet holistically. More and more vets are combining complementary treatments with standard veterinary care or are willing to refer you to a natural therapist who works with animals. This growth in complementary medicine in the animal world is partly due to demand by pet owners for a more holistic practice of animal care, and partly because vets themselves have found that modern drugs are not always the answer.

Many of the natural treatments detailed in this book have been around for hundreds, sometimes thousands, of years which is testimony to their curative powers. Animals have been treated by traditional means for as long as people have and, although complementary medicine may seem 'new', we are largely just re-discovering old systems of health care. Animals have always had an awareness of nature's medicinal powers and will look for edible plant cures in times of need.

In practice, natural medicine works in an holistic way which means it takes account of the animal's whole being, mind, body and spirit, and looks at all the different factors that are causing disease. In this way, treatment is directed at strengthening and supporting the total health of an animal and awakening its own powers of recovery. Rather than attacking the individual symptoms of disease, natural medicine aims to help the body to heal itself. This often involves permanent dietary and lifestyle changes for your pet. Without change, there can be no change!

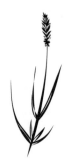

'Mammalian bodies are designed to live a healthy life, and the body has a tendency to make efforts to return to being healthy. So when you are looking at things holistically you are attempting to help the body to return to being healthy. You are also trying to remove the influences – medicinal, nutritional, or environmental – which are harmful and which lead to ill health.'

John Rohrbach, MVetMed, MRCVS

Both modern medicine and natural alternatives have a place in animal care. Sometimes drugs and surgery are the only way to save an animal's life, particularly in accident and emergency situations. Drugs can also help to 'buy time' while the more slow-acting natural treatments take hold. The important thing is to respect the strengths and weaknesses of both forms of medicine and to use whichever is the best for your pet. However, with less serious conditions, natural remedies support and strengthen the animal and, used correctly, do not have adverse side effects, which makes them a healthy alternative.

The emphasis of natural medicine has always been on prevention and, by taking time to re-assess your pet's diet, lifestyle and stresses, you can do a lot to improve their general health and reduce the chances of them becoming ill. For example, pets often mirror the state of mind of their owners, picking up on negative emotions around them, such as a pet living in a disharmonious household who may well become ill or start to display behavioural problems as a result, and often the whole household needs to take the same remedy as their pet!

There are lots of factors that contribute to disease, including pollution of our water, air and soil, chemical fertilisers and pesticides in farming, the additions of synthetic colourings, flavourings and preservatives in food, inadequate diet, stress, frequent or multiple vaccinations and genetic inheritance – the list is long! All these things stress the immune system and animals are just as vulnerable to these negative health factors as we are.

Unfortunately, one of the main characteristics of health care in developed countries is wanting instant answers and instant cures. In many ways we have become a quick-fix society and this rubs off onto our pets. They get given instant meals day after day and when they become ill, we do not consider that their diet and lifestyle might be the problem. Instead, we look for instant cures to heal them.

The impossible we do immediately, miracles take a little longer!

Many people want and expect miracle cures, but nature does not work like this. Natural medicine works with an animal's self-healing mechanism in a gentle way, bringing it back into balance and harmony. Always bear in mind the holistic nature of true healing and understand that disease is the result of a larger picture of lifestyle, diet and environmental factors. Giving natural remedies without changing other important factors may not cure your pet for long. The aim of this book is to encourage permanent healthy changes in your pet's life. For example, if your pet has cystitis you could use a homoeopathic remedy to clear it up – but it would be much better if you also changed the conditions that made it possible for the cystitis to occur in the first place. This might involve permanent changes in the diet and the regular addition of herbs, nutrients and other natural remedies which support the urinary tract and the immune system in fighting infections. There may also be emotional factors at play which are weakening the animal's resistance to disease and these can be healed with flower essences or healing. This is the true nature of holistic healing for animals.

A good diet is at the core of a healthy life and is the foundation of successful treatment. We need to take responsibility for our pet's health and general well-being. All the treatments and remedies in this book will be enhanced by a natural preservative-free diet, and in many cases dietary changes alone can

bring remarkable improvements in your pet's health. Many diseases suffered by cats and dogs these days can be avoided, including some of the chronic ones like heart disease, cancer and diabetes which have increased in line with our fast-food society.

The following chapters describe in detail the major holistic treatments for animals, how they work and what they can do to help. These include aromatherapy, acupuncture, biochemical tissues salts, chiropractic, diet and food supplements, flower essences, healing, herbs, homoeopathy and T-touch. Each chapter also tells you how to contact someone who can treat your pet and, where relevant, how to put together a natural remedies medicine chest for use at home.

Chapter 16 details remedies for first-aid use and Chapter 17 is an A–Z guide to specific ailments, treatments and remedies. Whichever remedies and treatments you decide to use, make sure you read the relevant chapters to get an understanding of what that treatment involves. This is especially important when carrying out the treatment yourself. Natural remedies are not meant to replace veterinary care for a seriously ill pet; however, many vets also practise complementary treatments and those that do not are often happy to refer you to somebody who does. When opting for natural treatments and remedies keep your vet informed of what you are doing.

Remember, prevention is better than cure.

CHAPTER TWO

Ten tips to keep your pet happy and healthy

Your pet needs…

1. Fresh air, sunshine and regular exercise. Dogs enjoy running around and sniffing out new smells, or just lying in the sun on a warm day. Cats are night-time creatures and love being outside at night, when they can hunt and prowl.

2. A healthy diet. A natural preservative-free diet is the best diet you can give your pet. They need fresh water every day, preferably filtered or bottled mineral water. Do not give snacks between meals because it encourages an animal to hang around constantly expecting food which can become irritating for you and makes them unable to settle.

3. Clear boundaries and adequate discipline. Pets need to know what they can and cannot do: which parts of the house or furniture they can use, what they can chew and what they cannot chew, and so on. Cats, especially ones that do not get out very much, need a scratching post or you may find your furniture serving the same purpose!

4. Their own bed, which should be warm and comfortable and made of natural fibres. Old wool blankets can be picked up cheaply in

charity shops and make great bedding material. Just like us, our pets sometimes want to have peace and quiet and need to have a place that is just for them. They also need enough rest.

5. Love and attention, companionship, touch. Most pets enjoy being touched by their owners, and it is therapeutic for them. It also shows them that you love them which makes for a contented animal.

6. Regular grooming and occasional bathing for dogs. Cats are natural groomers and rarely need a wash. Most dogs love to play in water, so take them to places where they can splash about and swim.

7. Play, such as chasing sticks, playing with toys, socialising with other animals. Animals enjoy interacting with their own kind and learning their own social hierarchy.

8. A job to do. This refers mainly to dogs. Some breeds are workers and need to be occupied doing jobs such as guarding, herding and racing. Bored animals can become disturbed and difficult.

9. Routine. Animals like a routine that they can rely on.

10. Being treated as an animal, not as a human being!

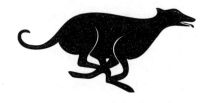

CHAPTER THREE

It's simple, isn't it?

- Pick up cat, and cradle as if holding a baby. Position forefinger and thumb on either side of cat's mouth and gently apply pressure to cheeks. As cat opens mouth, pop pill in. Allow cat to close mouth and swallow.
- Retrieve pill from floor, and cat from behind sofa. Repeat process.
- Retrieve cat from bedroom, throw soggy pill away. Take new pill from foil wrap. Cradle cat in left arm holding rear paws tightly with left hand. Force jaws open and push pill to back of mouth with right forefinger. Hold mouth shut for a count of 10.
- Retrieve pill from goldfish bowl and cat from top of wardrobe. Call spouse from garden. Kneel on floor with cat wedged firmly between knees, hold front and rear paws. Get spouse to hold head firmly with one hand while forcing wooden ruler into mouth. Drop pill down ruler and rub cat's throat vigorously.
- Retrieve cat from curtain rail, get another pill from foil wrap. Make note to repair curtains. Sweep shattered Doulton figures from hearth. Wrap cat in large towel with head just visible. Get spouse to hold cat and towel firmly under armpit. Put pill in end of drinking straw, force mouth open with pencil, and blow down drinking straw.
- Check to make sure pill not harmful to humans, drink glass of water

to take taste away. Apply bandage to spouse's forearm and remove blood from carpet with cold water and soap.

- Retrieve cat from neighbour's shed. Get another pill. Place cat in cupboard and close door onto neck with head showing. Force open mouth with desert spoon. Flick pill down throat with elastic band.

- Put door back on hinges. Ring fire brigade to retrieve cat from tree across the road. Take last pill from foil wrap. Tie cat's front paws to rear paws with garden twine and bind tightly to leg of dining table. Find heavy duty pruning gloves in shed, force cat's mouth open with small spanner. Push pill into mouth followed by a large piece of fillet steak and half a pint of water.

- Get spouse to drive you to casualty. Sit quietly while doctor stitches fingers and forearm and removes pill remnants from right eye. Call at furniture shop on way home to order new table.

- Go to the vet who puts cat on table. Cat lies there while vet pops open mouth and drops in pill. Cat swallows pill. Vet says: 'See how easy it is?'

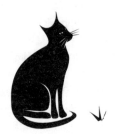

CHAPTER FOUR

A healthy diet

All healing begins with optimum nutrition

A healthy diet is the key to a healthy pet – which is why diet and food supplements are the first two subjects covered by this book. They are the most important contributions you can make to your pet's health – after all, feeding is the one thing you are able to influence for better or for worse. Animals on a natural, preservative-free diet rarely become ill because their bodies are better able to resist disease. The ultimate success of all of the treatments and remedies in the following chapters depends on a good diet.

> **Whatsoever was the father of disease, an ill diet was the mother.**
>
> *Chinese Proverb*

Just what is a healthy diet for dogs and cats? We are bombarded with so much information these days that it has become very confusing to know what is best for our pets. Is dried food better than tinned food? And what about the semi-moist foods, maybe they are better? Many people are scared not to buy commercially prepared 'complete' or 'balanced' foods in case they get it wrong and cause malnutrition in their pets. However, imagine bringing up a child solely on 'convenience foods' and expecting them to become a healthy, vibrant adult. We all know that fresh food is vital for good health, and that includes eating some of it raw. Commercially prepared pet foods are more or less 'convenience foods for pets' and most cats and dogs are fed tinned or dried food throughout their entire life. Pets, like people, need to eat real food.

A lot of health problems are food-orientated and you can do so much for your pet by making a few simple changes to their daily diet. Don't be scared to make your own pet food. After all, before the pet-food industry became an industry, everyone fed their dogs and cats real food – just ask your grandmother! Dogs and cats have been eating a fresh food, raw diet for thousands of years, so why do we suppose processed foods are better? The truth is, they're not. Cats and dogs do have specific requirements, but if you follow the advice given in this book on diet and supplements your pet will be much healthier in the long run.

Nutrition is the pivot upon which health and disease balance

Just as the number of people suffering from chronic diseases, such as arthritis, cancer, allergies, obesity, heart disease, skin problems and diabetes, is on the increase, so is the number of pets suffering similar problems. This increase of ill health goes hand in hand with the increase of processed and refined foods in the diet of both pets and people. In the case of your pet, some of the early warning signs of a poor-quality diet are a dull or smelly coat, skin problems, scratching, excess moulting, weight problems, bad breath, diarrhoea and constipation.

Good-quality food for your dog or cat is the key to preventing illness and is a vital factor in recovery. Whatever natural treatments or remedies you use, they will always be enhanced by a healthy, well-balanced diet. In fact, changing your pet's diet alone can produce spectacular improvements in their health and help them to avoid disease in the first place.

A healthy diet has a big impact on an animal's energy levels, appearance, performance and general health. This means making your pet's food from scratch, using fresh, wholesome ingredients with additional supplements.

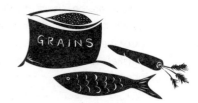

This is the best way to ensure a happy and healthy life.

The effects of a change of diet can be quite astonishing. Your pet may at last be free of a smelly skin, digestive problems, arthritis, obesity, behavioural problems and allergies. This is because a healthy, natural diet promotes the elimination of waste, reduces the intake of harmful substances, and increases an animal's resistance to disease.

Australian vet, Tom Lonsdale, has been campaigning to encourage his colleagues to urge their clients to feed their pets raw, meaty bones. Part of the campaign involves Tom standing for election as president of the Australian Veterinary Association. In a letter to his colleagues, he wrote (somewhat colourfully, but getting the message across):

'PLEASE DON'T VOTE FOR ME until you have conducted a thought experiment lasting at least one week.

During the week imagine eating canned stew and dry biscuits – nothing else. As the toxic sludge builds up you should neither brush your teeth nor chew on the furniture. Instead, ask a friend to brush your teeth once only for just two minutes.

As your mouth becomes progressively sore, cup your hands and smell your stinking breath and spare a thought. What must it be like for the millions of cats and dogs forced to live this way every day? Consider the potential, cruel consequences of chronic infection and immune compromise leading to multiple diseases and early death.

And then consider the evidence which I suggest demonstrates that the manufacturers of the *complete and balanced* formula, giving rise to the 85% prevalence of periodontal disease, immune compromise and widespread disease, have infiltrated the veterinary profession at every level. Notice that they appear to be in the universities, the laboratories, the surgeries and the associations, and then ask if this coincides with the interests of our profession or the animals under our care.

As the conclusion of your thought experiment, please cast your vote. It is my hope that of the 18,000 members of the Royal College of Veterinary Surgeons there are enough of us willing to make a difference to the current abominable state of affairs.

Thank you.'

Tom Lonsdale, BvetMed, MRCVS

Commercially prepared pet food

Pet food sits at the bottom of the pile as far as quality is concerned. As food generally becomes less healthy, for reasons such as modern farming practices, genetically modified foods, food processing etc, our pets are bearing the brunt. Ready-made pet foods vary hugely in quality and nutritional value. However, the nutritional analysis of the original ingredients is meaningless because commercially made pet foods are cooked and processed which, by definition, makes them deficient. While some are made from relatively good-quality ingredients, most contain poor-quality ingredients (some of which may horrify you!) and a host of harmful preservatives and additives. Not many people realise that it is quite legal to use diseased and contaminated meat in pet foods as well as the other animal parts that are passed unfit for human consumption. The exclusive use of commercially prepared pet food, with no additional fresh food, makes for an unbalanced and unhealthy diet.

**If *you* wouldn't eat dog or cat food, ask yourself why
you are happy to feed it to your *pet*.**

Chronic disease in our pets has been increasing in line with the use of commercially prepared pet foods. Most commercially made pet foods contain a host of unhealthy additives, colourings, flavouring and preservatives, sugar and salt, as well as other contaminants such as antibiotic residues and growth-hormone residues from meat, toxic metals, and agricultural chemical and pesticide residues. Toxins gather in the tissues and it is thought that the accumulative toxic effect of these can lead to all sorts of health problems, including liver and kidney disease, cancer, lowered immunity, skin problems, hair loss and behavioural problems, such as anxiety and aggression. High amounts of salt can lead to heart disease and kidney failure. High amounts of sugar can lead to diabetes, obesity, heart trouble and a long list of other health problems.

Commercially prepared pet foods are usually heat-treated which destroys a lot of the naturally occurring vitamins and enzymes. They also contain some of the primary allergens as their main ingredient – beef, wheat, dairy produce, corn, tuna-fish, and soya – which further stresses an animal's health.

Lead and other toxic metals contaminate pet foods as a result of processing and canning. They adversely affect the immune system and leave animals vulnerable to disease. An American Medical Association report cited that people who ate cat and dog food were in danger of consuming toxic levels of lead! Tuna-fish often contains high amounts of mercury and should therefore be avoided.

Tinned food

Most tinned cat and dog foods contain *meat* which may be labelled as 'meat derivatives' or 'meat by-products'. This is usually low quality and includes ears, horns, hooves, hides, beaks, feathers, entrails, high amounts of saturated fats, and diseased and cancerous meat that has been passed unfit for human consumption. In some countries, even dead pets and road kills find their way into pet food. Tinned food may also contain vegetable protein derived from cereals, texturised vegetable protein and soya, much of which are waste by-products of the human food industry, and again of suspect quality. Poor quality food offers substandard nutrition while, at the same time, taxes the liver, kidneys and digestive system as a whole.

Dried food

Dried foods have become increasingly popular because they are so convenient and don't smell as bad as tinned foods! You just open the packet, pour the right amount into the pet's bowl and that's that – no variety, no fresh meat, no fresh vegetables and often inadequate nutrition in the long term.

Dried foods are the subject of much controversy because they absorb so much fluid from the animal's digestive tract. Although dried-food manufacturers always recommend ensuring plenty of fresh water is available, you cannot be certain your pet will drink extra water to compensate. Try soaking some dried food overnight and see just how much water it takes up! If you do use a dried food, always soak it for at least half an hour to ensure your pet gets enough fluid. If they are not getting enough water to flush out metabolic wastes then kidney problems can result. Dried foods are also thought to contribute to kidney problems and cystitis due to their poor-quality protein content which upsets the body's acid/alkaline balance.

Most of the negative factors associated with tinned foods (see above) can also be attributed to dried food, with additional concern over the 'permitted' antioxidants. Reports from America suggest that some antioxidants may be related to a number of health problems, namely liver cancer, skin allergies, autoimmune diseases, and reproductive problems.

Semi-moist foods

Apart from the above, the additional problem with semi-moist food is the amount of sugar it contains, in some cases up to 25%! Animals can get addicted to sugar and become really picky about eating anything else. Sugar is a bringer of disease, sooner or later, including diabetes, allergies, cataracts, obesity, nervousness and tooth decay. Have you ever wondered how the semi-moist foods can last so long without needing to be kept in the fridge! Well, you've guessed it, the high sugar content acts as a preservative.

Dogs and cats often smell like the food they eat – if it isn't nice then it's time to change their diet!

Are all ready-made pet foods inadequate?

If you do have to use a ready-made pet food then look out for the following foods and try to avoid them: wheat, wheat gluten, dairy produce, soya, vegetable derivatives, vegetable by-products, cereals, beef, pork, artificial flavourings, colourings, preservatives, taste enhancers, added salt, sugar, meat by-products and meat derivatives.

The better-quality pet foods are generally free of the main food allergens. They tend to be made from brown rice, millet, lamb and poultry, and not from meat 'by-products' and 'substandard' grains. Just don't feed it every day if you wish to maximise your pet's health and well-being.

A natural preservative-free diet, made from fresh ingredients, is the best diet you can give to your pet, although there are times when a ready-made pet food makes life easier, such as if you are going away for the weekend or leaving your pet with somebody else for short periods of time. Whenever possible, it is best to make their diet from scratch and leave the convenience foods as a last resort. It is a question of doing the best that you can and getting into new ways and habits of preparing pet food.

What is a healthy diet for cats and dogs?

A variety of fresh, *real* food is the key to a healthy diet. Cats who only eat tuna, or dogs who only eat one kind of meat will eventually suffer health problems. The same goes for pets who are only fed processed food every day.

Cats are meat-eating animals (carnivores), therefore meat needs to form the bulk of their daily diet. They are designed to eat fresh, raw meat; however we have become so indoctrinated by the pet-food industry that only ready-made food is adequate, that we have forgotten that cats have dined on raw meat and bones for thousands of years. Think of all the birds and rodents they consume when out hunting at night. Cats are not vegetarian animals and need to be respected as such. Feed them raw meat and raw, meaty bones as the major ingredient of their diet, plus vegetables, fats and oils and, occasionally, grains.

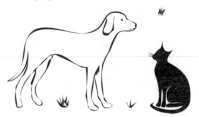

Dogs are not true carnivores, and are by nature scavengers and omnivorous. Because they have evolved to derive nutrients from a variety of sources it is easier to feed them a variety of foods – even fruit if they like it. For thousands of years, dogs have thrived on a varied diet of meat, bones, the contents of their prey's intestines, fruits, vegetables, grasses, nuts, seeds, berries, eggs and anything else they can find that's edible. A well-balanced, fresh, wholesome, preservative-free home-made diet is simple to prepare and often works out cheaper than ready-made pet foods. The main ingredients of your dog's diet should include meat and raw, meaty bones, fats and oils, vegetables and grains.

Protein
Meat Most meat is best served raw (or cooked as little as possible) since there is greater nutritional value in raw meat. Cats must have meat as their primary source of protein to get sufficient amounts of the amino acid, taurine, which is only found in meat and is essential to their well-being. Raw meat for cats and dogs is widely available from kennels, pet shops and most of the big pet superstores. It often comes frozen and guaranteed free of cereals, additives, preservatives, colourings, heads, feet and other low-grade animal parts. Always feed a variety of meat, such as chicken, turkey, tripe, lamb, beef, rabbit and fish. You can also buy fresh raw meat from your local butcher. The cheaper cuts are fine

for pets and try to include some organ meat once or twice a week: hearts, kidney, liver, lung or tripe. These can be cut up into bite-size pieces and given raw. Offal adds valuable trace minerals and vitamins to the diet. Pork should always be cooked.

If you are worried about bugs and bacteria in raw meat, remember that dogs and cats have sufficient stomach acid to deal with these; however as a preventative measure, you can add two or three drops of grapefruit-seed extract into their food (see Chapter 5).

Bones

Raw, meaty bones are an essential part of a cat's and dog's diet. They exercise the teeth and jaws and provide essential nutrients. Raw bones also act like a natural toothbrush and keep your pet's teeth strong and clean. The best ones for dogs and cats are marrow bones, chicken wings and necks, lambs bones, oxtails and rabbit carcasses. Again, variety is the key to a balanced diet.

Many people ask if raw bones are safe. Dogs and cats have been eating raw bones as part of their normal diet for millions of years. Cooked bones, on the other hand, may splinter and cause problems, and shouldn't be given to your pet, other than marrow bones which make great indoor toys. If your pet does not get bones regularly make sure you add bone-meal or a mineral supplement to their diet and give them something to chew on to exercise their jaws and keep their teeth healthy and strong.

Fish Dogs and cats enjoy fish, but be aware that it can be an allergy trigger. If you suspect an allergy to fish, then leave it out. Raw, frozen, minced fish can be bought from pet shops, kennels and pet superstores, or you can buy it fresh and feed it raw or lightly cooked. Tinned fish such as sardines, mackerel, pilchards can occasionally be used. Fish heads and tails make great stock and you can cook grains in it for extra flavour.

Eggs are a high-quality protein and can be added regularly to your pet's diet, preferably organic or free-range eggs.

Dairy produce Adult animals don't digest cow's milk very well; therefore it is best to avoid it. Yoghurt, cottage cheese and goat's milk are exceptions to this and can occasionally form some of the protein element of the diet. Also, raw, unpasteurised milk is acceptable in small amounts on an occasional basis.

Vegetable protein Vegetable protein can play a part in a dog's diet, although you must make sure it is always combined with a grain to make the protein content complete. Good sources include beans, lentils, soya mince, tofu, nuts, seeds, desiccated coconut.

How much protein?
Cats need more protein than dogs. The majority of a cat's diet should be made up of meat and/or meaty bones (at least 75%) with the addition of vegetables, grains (occasionally), fats and oils, herbs and supplements.

Dogs About 40–60% of a dog's diet needs to be made up of protein, including meaty bones, with the rest of the nutrients coming from grains, vegetables, fats and oils, herbs and supplements.

Fats and oils
Like humans, dogs and cats need substances found in fats and oils, called fatty acids. Two of these are essential, the omega 3 and omega 6 fatty acids, known as essential fatty acids, or EFAs. They are vital for normal functioning of the cells, tissues and organs. Generally, fats and oils are essential for a healthy, happy pet with a glossy coat and a healthy heart, skin and immune system. Many skin and coat problems indicate a lack of essential fats in the diet. They protect against splitting nails and claws, heart disease, hormone imbalances, cancer and diabetes. Dogs and cats need both saturated fats (animal fats) and unsaturated fats (vegetable and fish oils).

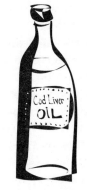

Saturated fats – Don't make the mistake of cutting out saturated fats entirely from your pet's diet because you think it is better for their health; they do need some, especially cats. Leftover bacon fat from cooking is a great way to add fat and flavour to your pet's food; other saturated fats include butter, beef dripping and meat fat.
Unsaturated fats/oils – These are as essential to life as vitamins and minerals and are found in fish and vegetable oils. The two most impor-

tant and well-known are the omega 3 and omega 6 essential fatty acids. Omega 3 EFAs are found in oily fish, fish liver and flaxseed/linseed oil. Omega 6 EFAs are found in vegetable oils, such as sunflower, safflower, evening primrose oil, and seeds, such as sesame, flaxseed, linseed and pumpkin. A daily dose of oil helps to prevent and treat a variety of health problems, such as fur balls in cats, feline acne, odour, drippy eyes and tear-stained faces. It improves dry and flaky skin, dandruff, eczema, oily skin and hot spots. Energy levels increase, mobility is greater, flea allergies heal quicker, digestive problems clear, inflammatory conditions improve.

Most oils are unstable and can go rancid quite quickly. They can become damaged by heat, air and light, so make sure you only buy good-quality, unrefined and cold-pressed oils. Keep them in the fridge and never heat them. (Olive oil is the most stable of the vegetable oils and can therefore be heated.)

Food sources: Fish, seeds, cold-pressed oils. If adding seeds to your pet's food, grind them up first to release the oil. Many of the good-quality supplements for dogs and cats include a balanced mix of EFAs within the formula, such as the Missing Link, Pet Plus. Higher Nature makes a balanced blend of EFAs for dogs and cats called Omegapet (see Chapter 5 for details).

How much?

Cats – 1/4 teaspoon of fish oil/fish-liver oil 2–3 times a week, plus 1/2 teaspoon of saturated fat 2–3 times a week.

Dogs – Up to 1 teaspoon of fish-liver oil 2–3 times a week, up to 1 table-spoon of vegetable oil 2–3 times a week. Occasionally add saturated fats.

Carbohydrates

These provide energy and fibre and include grains, vegetables and fruit.

Grains Fresh, whole, unrefined grains, such as brown rice, millet, oats, barley, and buckwheat are all good sources of carbohydrate and can be included in a dog's diet most days. All grains have to be cooked to open the starch granules so that they are more easily digested. The most important grain is brown rice, and this can be the staple carbohydrate of your pet's diet with other grains added for variety. Brown rice does take longer to cook than refined white rice; one of the easiest ways to cook it is to bring the pan to the boil, simmer for 15 minutes, then turn off the heat. As long as the lid is tightly fitting, the rice will have soaked up the water and be fully cooked by the time it has cooled.

All of the above grains are just as nutritious as wheat, but do not cause the common allergy problems associated with wheat. If you can get organic grains then this is always preferable. Brown rice is easy to digest and keeps the bowel healthy; oats contain iron and help cleanse the intestine; barley is a blood cleanser and good remedy for kidney and bladder problems.

How much?

Cats – Occasionally add grains to their food.

Dogs – Grains (and vegetables) can make up to 40–60% of a dog's diet.

Vegetables

These are an important addition to your pet's diet, providing additional vitamins, minerals and fibre. They can be given lightly cooked or raw. In the wild, cats and dogs would get much of their vegetable matter from eating the stomach contents of their prey, in an easy-to-digest form. Collect leftover vegetables or the bits you might normally throw away like potato peelings, the outside leaves of cabbage and lettuce, broccoli stalks and cauliflower leaves, and finely chop them up (food processors are good for this) and add them to your pet's meal. Cats will eat vegetables if they are chopped up small enough or pureed and mixed with something tasty. You can also cook potato peelings and vegetable ends with grains. Root vegetables, like carrots, parsnips and beetroot are best grated and added raw. Some vegetables have specific healing effects and can be added to your pet's diet depending on what is needed. Garlic, for example, cleanses the blood and prevents worms.

Raw, sprouted seeds are also a highly nutritious and vital food and can be added regularly to your pet's diet. They supply enzymes, vitamins and minerals. You can sprout seeds and grains yourself on a window sill or buy them ready-sprouted eg wheat, barley, mung beans, sunflower seeds, alfalfa.

How much?

Cats – Vegetables can make up to 25% of their daily diet.

Dogs – Vegetables (and grains) can make up to 40–60% of a dog's diet.

Fruit

Fruit adds vitamins, minerals and fibre to the diet. If your pet likes fruit it makes a healthy treat instead of the highly coloured and flavoured pet treats that are available. Fresh or dried fruit can be given, although dogs tend to like fruit more than cats. My own dog will happily eat a whole pear and will take them off the tree himself. My sister's dogs readily eat windfall apples and will 'climb' the plum trees to get at the ripe plums! Fruit, like vegetables, has specific therapeutic powers and can be added to the diet as necessary. Apricots, for example, are high in beta carotene which helps to protect against cancer; prunes alleviate consti-

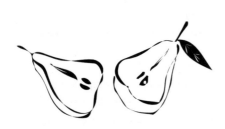

pation. You may have to cut them up really finely for cats and mix them in with their meal rather than feed them separately. Citrus fruits are not recommended as they are generally too acid for dogs and cats.

Why is raw food better?

Raw food contains many important elements that can be lost or destroyed by cooking, such as digestive enzymes, vitamins and minerals. Raw food is also 'alive' in that it is filled with life-force energy vital for good health, and for this reason alone it is important to feed your pet some food raw. Grains need to be cooked to make them digestible, but meat and vegetables have greater nutritional value when eaten raw or only very lightly cooked.

Treats

Fruit and vegetables make great treats, such as carrots, raisins, sultanas, and many pets will be just as happy with a raw carrot or a piece of apple as they would a less healthy alternative. Rice cakes and oatcakes are healthy alternatives to commercially made biscuit treats. There are also some commercially made pet treats made from lamb and rice and free from artificial additives which make good treats, or why not make your own – see later. Don't give animals chocolate or sweets as treats – it ruins their teeth, and chocolate is toxic to dogs.

Herbs

Culinary herbs like parsley, sage, mint, basil, lovage, thyme, oregano, marjoram, savory, and garlic can be added regularly to pet food. Animals will instinctively seek out herbs to eat in the wild. These can be used fresh or dried.

Leftovers

In times gone by, a dog and cat's diet would consist entirely of leftovers. Leftover food can be collected up and given to your pet at their next meal. Meaty leftovers are great for cats, and dogs will finish up almost any kind of food such as salad, vegetables, meaty scraps, baked-potato skins. Do not give them the unhealthy leftovers like puddings, pastries and sugary food though!

Changing to a new diet

It can sometimes take time to change to a new way of feeding your pet and getting into different routines and habits of cooking and shopping. It can take time for them to get used to new tastes and textures, especially if they have been used to diets high in sugar and salt. Some animals can become addicted to commercially prepared foods and to tuna-fish (which can also have a dangerously high mercury content). Just persevere until they come round. Sometimes fasting a healthy animal for a day or two helps to heighten their hunger for new and different foods and breaks a habit of finicky eating! One of the best ways of changing their diet is to introduce the new food gradually and phase out the old food at the same time. You might want to do this over a week or two. Pet owners often notice changes in their pet following a change to a natural diet; healthier coats, better teeth, stronger bones, fewer infections, fewer problems with fleas and other parasites – and far less wind!

Make it fun!

Cooking for your pet need not be a chore and it is fun to try new recipes now and again. As your pet's health improves you may find yourself following some of the same healthy principles!

How many meals a day?

A healthy adult cat or dog in general only needs one meal per day, although puppies, kittens and older pets will need to have several small meals spread throughout the day. There are no hard and fast rules about when is the best time to feed your pet and usually you will find a time that suits you and your pet. The most important thing is that meal times are regular.

How much food?

Animals differ in their needs, so the best way to work out how much food your pet needs is to use a common-sense approach – if they gain weight, then cut down on their food; and if they lose weight, add more. So much depends on their daily activity, age, breed and other individual influences. Excessive weight gain or weight loss could be a sign of a serious illness, and in this case it would be advisable to take your pet to the vet.

Elderly pets, puppies and kittens have different nutritional needs and this will be covered later in this chapter. For feeding guidelines for pregnant animals, see Chapter 17.

Feeding dos and don'ts

- Feed at the same time every day.
- Take the food away after half an hour if they have not eaten it all. (This includes cats whose food is often left all day for them to pick at.) In the wild, cats and dogs would not have a constant source of food to pick at throughout the day and periods of fasting between meals are very important for efficient digestion and detoxification.
- Fresh water should be available at all times, preferably filtered or bottled water.
- Do not feed from the table or give too many treats.
- Food and water bowls should be made from glass, stainless steel or porcelain.
- Cook food in stainless-steel pans, not aluminium or copper pans.

Is a natural diet always the best choice for my pet?

A natural diet is the first choice for most, but not all, pets. Some dogs and cats with low energy systems aren't able to tolerate the energy in natural foods and may fare better by continuing to eat processed foods.

However it's worth remembering that this is the result of long-term feeding of processed foods and other contributory factors, such as multiple or frequent vaccinations, so that the animal's system has become too weak to cope with a natural diet! This may be the case with elderly pets.

Allergies

(See also Digestive problems and Allergies in Chapter 17.) Allergies and allergy-based diseases are becoming more frequent in pets and inadequate diet is thought to be one of the main contributing factors. Symptoms of allergy can be many and varied, but some common ones include sneezing, scratching, fur loss, reactions to flea bites, diarrhoea and constipation. Behavioural problems too are associated with allergies – just like children, pets are sensitive to E numbers! Colourings are not put in food for an animal's benefit and are totally unnecessary. Allergic reactions can be caused by environmental elements too, like house dust, house-dust mites and pollens. A poor or inadequate diet impairs the digestive system and damages the immune system to the point that it cannot function properly and becomes oversensitive.

Common trigger foods

These include beef, pork, cow's milk, corn, wheat and wheat gluten, eggs, soya, yeast and tuna-fish.

Commercially prepared foods use some of the primary allergens as their main ingredients. The damaging effects will be much worse if these foods are also full of artificial dyes, preservatives, sugar, salt, and flavourings.

What do I feed an allergic pet?

First cut out all the possible allergens from their diet and environment. A one-day fast is helpful in clearing the system of toxins (see Fasting dos and don'ts) and then reintroduce food, starting with ones that are not usually a problem, like brown rice and lamb. Grated carrots can also be added to their meal along with fats and oils. Stick to this for at least a week with no other type of food and see if your pet's symptoms and general health improves. After a week you can begin to reintroduce new foods one day at a time and watch to see if they cause any adverse reactions. If not, you can be fairly sure that they can tolerate that new food and it can become part of the whole diet. Any food that does cause an adverse reaction should be omitted. When allergies are suspected, it is best to give your pet bottled or filtered water, rather than tap water, and organic food.

Supplements for an allergic pet

The most likely allergic trigger is brewer's yeast or a yeast-based B vitamin or multi-vitamin complex. If yeast is a problem, look for yeast-free supplements. Many of the cat and dog multi-minerals and vitamins are also free of other possible allergenic substances such as dairy, sugar, soya, gluten, corn, wheat, egg, artificial colourings and flavourings, so look out for these. Whether your pet is allergic or not, it is always advisable to use the better-quality supplements. Adding digestive enzymes and probiotics helps in cases of allergy (see Chapter 5 for supplementing your pet's diet).

Feeding an elderly pet

Older pets have different dietary needs than younger animals. As dogs and cats age, their bodily functions can become less efficient, particularly in digesting food and eliminating waste products. They are also prone to putting on weight as they become less active. If your pet is gaining weight then reduce their food until you reach the optimum dietary amount for them.

An elderly pet's diet needs to be easy to digest and of good-quality ingredients.

The protein content of the diet of both cats and dogs should be moderately reduced to lessen the eliminative load on the kidneys, but make sure it is high-quality protein.

Add plenty of fibre to avoid constipation, such as brown rice, raw vegetables and psyllium husks.

Many older pets also need digestive enzymes and other dietary supplements added regularly to their food to ensure optimum nutrition. (See Chapter 5.)

To help with digestion, feed elderly pets on a little-and-often basis, rather than just one large meal in a day.

Feeding puppies and kittens

The healthier a young animal's diet is when they are growing, the better their overall health will be throughout their life. After weaning, a natural, preservative-free diet is the best start you can give any young pet, and it helps to reduce the risk of allergies and behavioural problems from arising. A good diet will help the immune system to grow strong and protect them from disease.

The first six months are a time of rapid growth, and puppies and kittens may need twice as much food as their parents. They will also need to be fed at least three times a day. Little and often is the best way to feed young animals. Puppies and kittens also need a higher percentage of protein and fat in their diet than adult dogs and cats. Their food can be enriched with egg yolks, honey, molasses, cod-liver oil, brewer's yeast and vitamin C. Raw garlic or garlic capsules added to their food daily will help protect them from worms and other parasites (see Chapter 5 for food supplements).

Also give them plenty of raw, meaty bones to chew on. This not only builds strong, healthy teeth, but keeps them occupied in a most natural way.

After six months, they only need to be fed twice a day, and then just once a day after nine months.

Home-made treats for dogs and cats

Dog/cat biscuits

2 tablespoons bran/bran flakes (eg wheat, oat, or rye)
2 cups wholemeal flour (eg wheat, rice, rye, etc)
1 heaped tablespoon brewer's yeast (if no yeast allergy), or crushed vitamin B complex tablets
1 cup wheat germ
2 teaspoons blackstrap molasses (1 teaspoon for cats)
1 tablespoon vegetable oil
30g butter (cats)
1 teaspoon fish-liver oil (cats)
Water

Mix all the ingredients together in a bowl and add enough water to make a firm dough. Shape the dough into small, flat biscuit shapes and bake in a moderate oven for about half an hour or until dry and hard. The biscuits will keep for at least a week if stored in a cool, dry, airtight container. All the above ingredients can be bought in health-food stores. (Substitute wheat bran and wheat flour for an alternative grain if you suspect an allergy to wheat.)

These make a really healthy biscuit and are also a fun treat for children to make for their pets.

An ill pet

Never force an ill animal to eat; dogs and cats will naturally fast when they are feeling unwell. Always make sure that plenty of fresh water is available.

Fasting

Fasting is one of the best ways to detoxify the body and stimulate healing. When energy is not being used up on digestive processes, the body can concentrate on repair, renewal and fighting disease. Fasting is particularly effective in healing infections, fevers, skin problems and digestive disorders. Animals in the wild will naturally fast when they are ill, and so will many domestic pets. Regular fasting of healthy animals will bring enormous health benefits and help to boost their immune system and keep their body free of harmful toxins. Some animals do this naturally on a weekly basis, and you may wish to try introducing regular, one-day fasts.

Fasting dos and don'ts

- Never fast a pet that is young, old, pregnant, lactating or ill, without veterinary supervision. Healthy, mature pets can fast for a full day on a regular basis but no more than one day a week.
- During a fast you can give your pet liquid nourishment such as:
  Home-made barley water, with or without honey added to it. This is rich in magnesium and helps ease rheumatism and skin complaints, and purifies the blood. Simmer one tablespoon of pearl barley in fresh water for 20 minutes, cool and strain.
  Home-made rice water. Simmer one tablespoon of brown rice in water for 40 minutes, strain and cool. You can add fenugreek seeds for added (curry) flavour.
  Vegetable or chicken broth (the strained liquid only). Use a mixture of root vegetable, onions, garlic, potato peelings and/or chicken bones simmered in water.

Water and apple cider vinegar (plus honey if desired).
Fish-head broth (strained liquid only).
Stock made from meat bones (strained liquid only).
Freshly made vegetable juice.
Aloe vera juice diluted with water – a wonderful detoxifier.

- Dogs and cats can also be given raw bones on a fast day.
- Leave out any additional vitamins and minerals while fasting.
- Make sure your pet gets plenty of fresh air and light exercise.
- Give them lots of affection during a fast so they don't feel you have just forgotten to feed them!
- It is a good time to give them a bath with a natural, herbal shampoo especially if they have skin or coat problems.
- End the fast slowly with a small meal of wholesome ingredients.

When an ill animal does want food again then one of the most beneficial things you can do is to change their diet to a natural, home-made, preservative-free one plus supplements.

Useful Information

Canine Health Concern
PO Box 1, Longnor, Derbyshire SK17 0JD (UK)
Tel: 07071 226482
E-mail: K9Health@aol.com
Internet discussion group, send a blank e-mail to:
K9health-subscribe@egroups.com
Internet: http://members.aol.com/k9health/wwwk9h/index.htm
(CHC provides information on preventative health care for dogs and cats, including natural diet, homoeopathic alternatives to vaccination, seminars, courses and quarterly newsletter)
Tom Lonsdale's website: www.rawmeatybones.com

CHAPTER FIVE

Food supplements

The question of whether food supplements are necessary is a much debated point. Dogs and cats eating a well-balanced, fresh-food diet may not need much in the way of supplements. However, there may be times of extra need such as illness, growth, pregnancy, lactation and for elderly animals. Many people think there is no need to supplement their pet's diet if they are feeding them a commercially prepared 'balanced' or 'complete' food, however this is not the case.

Generally, there would be less need for supplements if our food contained everything that we and our pets require; however, modern farming methods and the use of chemicals deplete the soil of essential nutrients and consequently our food is depleted. Food processing further depletes food of valuable nutrients and enzymes, and the addition of synthetic additives and preservatives increases the need for supplementation yet more.

All animals are different and have individual needs. Some may need extra supplements every day, particularly if they work or exercise hard, whilst others may only need extra supplements in times of special need. However, by adding food supplements on a regular basis to your pet's diet you will improve their health and protect them from illness.

Vitamins and minerals can make a dramatic difference to the health of dogs and cats. They can also be powerful tools in treating disease.

Vitamins

Vitamins are vital to health and they regulate body processes. They are easily destroyed by cooking and food processing, and therefore need to be added to the diet if your pet eats processed food.

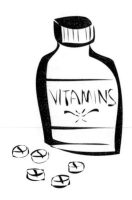

Vitamin A is vital for healthy eyes and good eyesight and is important for maintaining strong bones and healthy skin, coat, teeth and gums. Vitamin A is also a powerful antioxidant which protects the body's cells and tissues from pollution damage and cancer. It also has immune-system-enhancing properties, and is particularly good for healing respiratory problems, and is vital for the development and growth of kittens and puppies. Too much vitamin A can be toxic, so it is always best to use food sources of vitamin A or supplement it as part of a balanced vitamin complex.

Food sources: Fish-liver oil, liver, and eggs. The easiest way to supplement vitamin A is by adding fish-liver oil to the diet.

How much? Up to 1 teaspoon of fish-liver oil weekly for cats, up to 3 teaspoons weekly for dogs. If you are already giving a multi-vitamin complex beware of overdosing with vitamins A by adding liver or fish-liver oil to the diet as well. Remember that animal liver is also high in vitamin A.

The **B vitamins** are essential for healthy organs and nervous system, a glossy coat and healthy skin. Some of the B vitamins are needed for red-blood-cell formation. They help to keep parasites at bay, protect your pet from stress and boost the immune system. B vitamins are unlikely to be overdosed since they are water soluble and any excess is naturally eliminated by the body.

Food sources: Wholegrains, meat, eggs and brewer's yeast. Or you can use a yeast-free vitamin-B complex if your pet is allergic to yeast.

How much? Up to 1/2 teaspoon brewer's yeast for cats daily, up to 1 tablespoon daily for dogs sprinkled on their food. Cats and dogs generally love the taste of brewer's yeast. If they do have an allergy to yeast, buy a yeast-free vitamin-B complex and reduce the human recommended amount to suit the size of your pet.

Vitamin C is vital for healing cuts and wounds and internally damaged tissues. It keeps the immune system healthy, protects against infection and cancer, and encourages healthy skin, bones, cartilage, teeth and gums. It is also a major detoxifier, including toxic metals. Although dogs and cats can make their own vitamin C, if their diet is inadequate or their health impaired then their ability to make adequate amounts of vitamin C will also be impaired. Pet foods do not contain additional vitamin C because it is thought that dogs and cats can make enough in their bodies. It has been found to be a preventive against hip dysplasia, lameness, arthritis, viral diseases and skin problems. A sick animal will have a great need for vitamin C and can be given large quantities up to the point of bowel tolerance. This is the point at which too much vitamin C will cause diarrhoea, but it is a very good guide to how much your pet's body is needing.

Food sources: Green, leafy vegetables, potatoes, cauliflower, nettles, parsley. Vitamin C powder can be sprinkled into food, or given in capsule form.

How much? On a daily basis cats can have up to 500mg and dogs 500–7,000mg depending on their size. See specific ailments and treatments for times of increased need such as illness, infections and wound-healing.

Vitamin D is needed for the absorption of other nutrients such as calcium and phosphorus and is therefore essential in helping to maintain bone structure and healthy teeth. Like vitamin A, vitamin D can be toxic in large doses.

Food sources: Eggs, oily fish, sunlight. Fish-liver oil is a good way to supplement both vitamins A and D. Reduce the amount of vitamin D during the summer months when animals are getting more sunlight.

How much? The best way to supplement vitamin D is with fish-liver oil: 1/2 teaspoon for cats, 1–2 teaspoons for dogs, once or twice a week or as part of a multi-vitamin complex.

Vitamin E is a potent antioxidant that protects animals against pollution damage and cancer. Vitamin E enhances the beneficial effect of vitamin A.

It also plays an important role in a healthy reproductive system and efficient lactation, a healthy heart and good circulation. It aids wound healing and can be used externally to promote skin healing. It also prevents fats from going rancid. Rancid fats are one of the worst known cancer-causing agents.

Food sources: Wheat-germ oil, wheat germ, vegetable oils, whole grains, leafy greens and organ meats. Vitamin E is also available in capsule form.

How much? Up to 50–100iu daily for cats, up to 400iu daily for dogs depending on their size.

Multi-vitamins are a simple and practical way of ensuring that your pet is getting a basic level of these essential nutrients. There are many good quality ones available designed for cats and dogs appropriately balanced for their different needs (see Where to buy food supplements at the end of the chapter). Or you can make your own food supplement – see later.

Minerals

Minerals are important for growth and development but they are often deficient in a pet's diet. Some minerals (like calcium and magnesium) are needed in large quantities, while others (like zinc and selenium) are just needed in tiny amounts.

Calcium is essential for healthy bones and teeth as well as keeping the nerves, heart and muscles healthy. Growing puppies and kittens, pregnant females and lactating mothers have a special need for calcium in the diet.

Food sources: Bone-meal, raw, meaty bones, sardines, green, leafy vegetables, seaweeds. One of the best ways to supplement calcium is with raw, meaty bones.

How much? Pets who are regularly getting bones may not need additional calcium except in times of specific need such as pregnancy and growth. For pets not getting raw, meaty bones, give sardines weekly or give 1/4 teaspoon of bone-meal for cats daily, up to 1 teaspoon daily for dogs.

Iron is vital for healthy blood, and deficiency can lead to anaemia. Vitamin C increases the uptake of iron in the body.

Food sources: Offal, meat, sardines, egg yolks, dark green leafy vegetables, dried fruit, and the herbs nettle and parsley.

How much? 5mg daily for cats, up to 15mg daily for dogs. Iron is usually included in a multi-mineral complex and can be added separately in times of specific need.

Magnesium is important for healthy bones and teeth, nerve and muscle function. Magnesium is also a great pain reliever and calmative, along with calcium.
Food sources: Wholegrains, dried figs, green, leafy vegetables, pulses.
How much? There may not be adequate amounts of magnesium in the diet (due to depleted amounts in the soil) especially in times of specific need. A multi-mineral complex for cats and dogs will usually contain magnesium. Epsom salts are also a good source of magnesium – add a pinch daily to a cat's food or 2–3 pinches for a dog.

Potassium and sodium are synergistic and need to be kept in balance. Some pet foods have added salt which is unnecessary and can lead to health problems. The two minerals work together to maintain fluid and electrolyte balance in the cells and tissues. Potassium helps to regulate blood pressure and maintain a normal heartbeat. Ready-made pet foods tend to be low in potassium and high in sodium.
Food sources: potassium – Dandelions, bananas, avocados, leafy vegetables and garlic. Apple cider vinegar adds potassium to the diet and is one of the easiest ways to supplement it; *sodium* – Celery, kelp, sea salt.
How much? There is rarely a need to add sodium to the diet. For additional potassium, add 1 teaspoon of apple cider vinegar to each pint of water for both cats and dogs, or add it to their food; 1/2 teaspoon for cats, and up to 6 teaspoons for dogs.

Zinc is vital for normal growth, the development and health of the reproductive system, the proper functioning of the immune system, healing cuts and wounds and for maintaining a healthy skin and coat.
Food sources: Meat, poultry, eggs, shellfish, pumpkin seeds and butter-beans.
How much? 5mg for cats, up to 15mg daily for dogs. Zinc is best supplemented as part of a multi-mineral complex and added separately in times of extra need.

Don't panic, you don't have to add these things every day to your pet's food! A good quality multi-vitamin and mineral complex will supply most or all beneficial supplements. As mentioned before, there may be times of specific need when extra nutrients will be required. The above is a guide to how to improve your pet's diet in the way that you and they find most suitable. Multi-vitamins and minerals are a convenient way to ensure a balanced amount of the important nutrients for your pet. Some of the best-quality all-in-one supplements for dogs and cats include: The Missing Link, Pet Plus, Barley Dog and Barley Cat, Pet Essentials and Juice Plus for pets (see Where to buy food supplements at the end of the chapter), or you can make your own – see later. During times of specific need you may wish to add specific vitamins and minerals such as iron for anaemia or zinc and vitamin C to fight infection and to heal skin problems. For specific ailments and treatments, see Chapter 17.

Giving capsules and tablets

Many of the ready-made supplement formulas come in powder form, but if you are using capsules or tablets and you find that your pet won't take them, try opening the capsules up and sprinkling the contents into their food or mixing the contents with a small amount of something they love. Tablets can be crushed and mixed in with food or a tasty treat like butter, fish paste, molasses or sardines. Always give your pet an affectionate pat or a treat if they have managed to swallow something they have earlier resisted.

Other valuable supplements

Aloe vera juice is a great detoxifier, bowel cleanser, digestive aid and immune-system booster. It can be added to food or water. (Avoid if your pet is pregnant.)

Apple cider vinegar adds potassium to the diet and is helpful in treating arthritis. It also helps the body to absorb minerals better. It is an old, folk remedy which is claimed to improve health, reduce infection and aid digestion and bowel function. It also helps to keep the pH balance right in the gut.

How much? Add 1 teaspoon per pint of water to your cat's or dog's drinking water, or add it to their food: 1/2 teaspoon for cats, up to 6 teaspoons for dogs.

Bone-meal provides calcium and other minerals to the diet. In the wild, animals eat the bones as well as the flesh of animals which naturally balances the high phosphorus content of meat with the high calcium content of the bones.
How much? 1/4 teaspoon bone-meal daily for cats and up to 1 teaspoon daily for dogs.

Brewer's yeast is one of the best sources of the whole range of B vitamins and cats and dogs love the taste. It also provides some protein.
How much? 1/4–1/2 teaspoon daily for cats, up to one tablespoon for dogs.

Digestive enzymes enhance the absorption and digestion of food and are useful for older animals, pets with allergies or those in need of digestive support, especially during illness and recovery.
How much? Usually 1 to 2 capsules with each meal, or a 1/2 to 1 teaspoon of powdered enzymes. Acorn Supplements Ltd (UK) make a combined enzyme and probiotic formula called Pet Plus which is an ideal digestive support for pets recovering from illness, following a course of antibiotics (which can destroy the friendly intestinal flora), after surgery, for elderly pets or those with digestive upsets.

Evening primrose oil is high in omega 6 essential fatty acids and has anti-inflammatory and immune-boosting properties and helps to balance the hormones and keep the skin healhty. A good oil to add if your pet has allergies, skin complaints, diabetes, autoimmune disorders, hormone imbalance.
How much? 1–2 capsules daily with food.

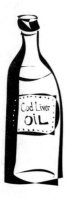

Fish-liver oil/Cod-liver oil is a good source of vitamins A and D as well as adding fish oil to the diet which helps to maintain a healthy heart and circulatory system, they keep the skin and coat healthy. Give 1/4 teaspoon 2 to 3 times a week for cats, up to 1 teaspoon 2 to 3 times a week for dogs.

Garlic has a range of health giving properties including being an effective anti-viral, anti-bacterial and anti-fungal agent. It fights infections, expels worms and parasites and assists in the healing process to name just a few of its health-giving actions.

How much? 1/4 clove raw garlic daily for cats, 1/2 –1 clove daily for dogs mixed in with their meal. Garlic capsules are available if they do not like the taste of it raw. Don't use deodorised ones, since they aren't as potent. Give one capsule every few days for cats, 1 or 2 capsules a day for dogs.

Green super-foods, such as barley grass and spirulina, provide a wealth of essential nutrients, often lacking in conventional foods grown in depleted soils, and further depleted by food processing. Green foods keep an animal's body alkaline and less prone to disease. They are a rich source of chlorophyll which keeps the body detoxified and energised. Animals instinctively eat green foods to obtain a wide range of valuable nutrients and to defend themselves against disease.

Sources: Wheat grass, barley grass, alfalfa, and the algae, chlorella and spirulina. They can be bought powdered or as tablets and capsules.

How much? Up to 1/2 teaspoon powdered greens daily for cats, up to 3 teaspoons daily for dogs.

Glucosamine sulphate is a naturally occurring substance found in joint cartilage and is obtained from the exoskeletons of marine animals (shrimps, crabs and lobsters). It helps to rebuild cartilage and repair damaged joints, tendons and ligaments. It also helps to reduce inflammation and relieve pain. In double blind studies, glucosamine sulphate has been shown to yield as good or even better results than medical, non-steroid anti-inflammatories, which makes it an important supplement for musculo-skeletal problems.

How much? Give 500–1,000mg, 2 or 3 times daily for at least 2 months, after which you can reduce the dose.

Grapefruit-seed extract is a potent healing tool and has been described as 'the world's smallest medicine chest'. It can inactivate viruses, yeasts, fungi, bacteria, parasites and worms. It is powerfully effective against a broad spectrum of germs and bacteria but is non-toxic and non-weakening to the immune system – unlike pharmaceutical antibiotics. It is naturally derived, has little or no adverse effect on the beneficial gut bacteria, making it a highly effective treatment for a range of digestive problems, from diarrhoea to parasites. Grapefruit-seed extract can be used internally and externally.

Internal use – Add 5–15 drops (depending on the size of the animal) to food and give 2 or 3 times daily. Add a couple of drops on a toothbrush to clean your pet's teeth. Grapefruit-seed extract can also be bought in capsule form. One capsule is equivalent to 15 drops.

External use – Dilute 10 drops in an eggcup of water or oil. You can also fill a small spray bottle with grapefruit-seed extract and water for a potent antibiotic spray.

Honey is good for the immune system and eases digestive problems. It adds important nutrients to the diet and is a useful addition to a liquid fast. Honey is a natural energiser. It can also be used externally to heal burns.

Kelp is another rich source of vitamins (especially the B vitamins) and minerals (especially potassium and iodine) and helps to promote a shiny coat and a healthy skin. As it is also a good source of iodine it supports thyroid function and regulates metabolism. It can be bought dried and cooked with a grain or used in powdered form added to food.

How much? 1/4 teaspoon daily for cats, up to 1 teaspoon daily for dogs. You can also add sea vegetables to your pet's food, such as nori, kombu, wakame and dulse.

Lecithin granules are a fat emulsifier and help to keep cholesterol and fatty deposits from forming in the body. Lecithin is good for older pets and helps to metabolise fats.

How much? Lecithin granules can be bought in health-food shops and can be sprinkled on food. 1/4 teaspoon daily for cats, up to 1 teaspoon daily for dogs.

Probiotics (such as Lactobacillus acidophilus) are friendly intestinal bacteria and are vital for good health. These friendly bacteria inhabit the intestinal system of all animals. Probiotics help pets absorb nutrients, boost the immune system, keep the pH balance of the gut right and eliminate toxins. Always give your pet probiotics following a course of antibiotics, which tend to wipe out both the unfriendly and the friendly bacteria. Any digestive disturbance like diarrhoea or constipation will benefit from acidophilus. Live yoghurt is also a good source of the

friendly bacteria. Probiotics are widely available in health-food stores. Store in the fridge.
How much? 1 capsule/1/4 teaspoon powder daily for cats, 2 capsules/ 1/2 teaspoon powder for dogs.

Psyllium husks are a form of natural vegetable fibre and are brilliant for cleansing the bowel and carrying toxins out of the body. They will help to alleviate a constipated pet and maintain bowel health.
How much? Psyllium husks come in capsules or as loose powder which can be sprinkled in food. 1/2 teaspoon daily for cats, up to 2 teaspoons daily for dogs, as required.

Wheat-germ oil is a great source of vitamin E.
How much? One capsule daily for cats, up to 4 capsules daily for dogs.

A basic home-made supplement for cats and dogs

Mix together the following ingredients and store in an airtight container in the fridge.

1/2 cup	Powdered green super-food eg Alfalfa, wheat/barley grass, chlorella, spirulina
1/4 cup	Powdered kelp
1/4 cup	Desiccated coconut
1/2 cup	Ground mixed seeds – hemp, linseed/flaxseed, sunflower
1/4 cup	Pumpkin seeds (whole)
1/4 cup	Powdered probiotics
1/2 cup	Psyllium husks
1/4 cup	Lecithin granules
1/2 cup	Brewer's yeast (not for pets allergic to yeast or suffering from yeast infections)
1/4 cup	Dried herbs – dandelion, nettle, parsley and oregano
1/4 cup	Wheat germ

Optional:

1/2 cup	Bone-meal powder (if your pet is not getting raw, meaty bones)

A coffee grinder is ideal for grinding up dried herbs and seeds. You will be able to get most of the above ingredients in your local health-food store.

How much? Up to 2 teaspoons per day for cats, up to 6 teaspoons per day for dogs.

Useful information

Where to buy food supplements
Pet shops, pet superstores and health-food shops will have many of the supplements listed above. However specialist suppliers of food supplements for pets are listed below:

UK
Acorn Supplements Ltd
PO Box 103, Robertsbridge, East Sussex TN32 5ZT
Tel: 01580 881333 Fax: 01580 881444
Email: acorn-orders@europe.com
Internet: www.acorn.uk100.com
(Suppliers of an excellent range of high-quality, natural-food supplements and products for dogs and cats, including The Missing Link, Pet Plus, Osteo-Ease, Immune Plus, grapefruit-seed extract products, Natural De-Wormer, Flea Clear, Beyond Greens. Also homoeopathic and herbal remedies and Bach flower remedies.)

Higher Nature
Burwash Common, East Sussex TN19 7LX
Tel: 01435 882880
Fax: 01435 883720
(Suppliers of Omegapet, Glucosamine Plus, Animal Aloe, and other natural supplements for dogs and cats.)

Savant Distribution Ltd
7 Wayland Croft, Adel, Leeds LS16 8LA
Tel: 0113 230 1993
Email: info@savant-health.com
Internet: www.savant-health.com
(Suppliers of high-quality, natural and organic food supplements for animals – including The Missing Link, Pet Essentials and cold pressed oils.)

All Seasons Health
19-21 Victoria Road North, Southsea, Hampshire PO5 1PL
Tel/Fax: 01705 755660
Email: info@allseasons.demon.co.uk
Internet: www.earthrise.com
(Great source of natural, green-food nutritional supplements, organi-
cally grown, gathered from around the world.)

Faithful Friends
43 New Road, Broomfield, Chelmsford, Essex CM1 7AN
Tel/Fax: 01245 443372
(Suppliers of a range of natural remedies and products for cats and
dogs, including herbal and homoeopathic remedies, aromatherapy
products and magnetic collars.)

Ireland
The Aisling Foundation
Dunnamark Falls, Bantry, Co. Cork
Tel: 027 51567
Fax: 027 52052
Email: grapefruit@tinet.ie
(Suppliers of grapefruit-seed extract – liquid and capsule form.)

US
Earth Animal
606 Post Road East, Westport, CT 06880
Tel: (800) 622 0260
(Offers a complete line of natural products for dogs and cats, including
nutritional supplements, flea and tick prevention products, and shampoos.
Mail order service also available.)

Dr Goodpet
PO Box 4547, Inglewood, CA 90309
Tel: (800) 222 9932
(Suppliers of nutritional supplements, shampoos, homoeopathics etc.
Mail order service available.)

Pat McKay, Inc
396 W Washington Blvd, Ste 600, Pasadena, CA 91103
Tel: 1-800-975-7555 or 626-296-1120
Fax: 626-296-1126
Email: patmckay@gte.net
Internet: www.home1.gte/patmckay
(Frozen, raw foods, nutritional supplements, books.)

Earthrise Nutriceuticals
424 Payram Street, Petaluma, California 94952
Tel: (707) 778-9078
Fax: (707) 778-9028
Email: info@earthrise.com
Internet: www.earthrise.com
(Suppliers of organically grown, certified pesticide-free, super-green foods.)

Pines International
PO Box 1107, Lawrence, Kansas 6604-8107
Tel: (785) 841-6016
Fax: (785) 841 1252
Email: info@wheatgrass.com
Internet: www.wheatgrass.com
(Suppliers of super-green foods, organically grown, certified pesticide-free.)

CHAPTER SIX

Vaccinations

The issue of giving routine and annual vaccinations is a hot potato and can leave many pet owners confused and bewildered about what is best for their pet. Opinion about vaccines is as divided and emotive in the pet world as it is in the human world. There is much debate about whether vaccines can, in fact, be harmful in the long run and recent evidence suggests that AIDS emerged as a direct result of contaminated polio vaccines. The whole issue of immunisation needs to be given objective evaluation and re-evaluation.

There are many questions we pet owners need to ask, such as, do immunisation programs really protect to anything like the degree that is claimed? Are the short- and long-term side effects a reasonable price to pay for the possible protective benefits? Are there alternative ways of achieving protection from infectious diseases without adverse side effects?

> 'I think that vaccines, justly credited as the tamers of disease epidemics, are nevertheless the leading killers of dogs and cats in America today.'
>
> *Martin Goldstein, DVM*

Many parents are convinced there is a link between their child's autism and vaccinations and many pet owners too are now beginning to link their pet's disease symptoms with immunisation. Despite the huge body of evidence in support of conventional vaccines for dogs and cats, there is also mounting evidence against the routine administration of vaccines. Many homoeopathic vets feel that routine, annual vaccination can lead to disease reactions and a breakdown of the animal's immune system. Others suggest there is a strong connection between vaccination and behavioural problems. In America, the veterinary immunologists claim that vaccinations need only to be given once or twice during an animal's lifetime. In the UK pet owners are asked to follow a program of annual vaccinations, although it's known that the protective effects of the vaccines last for many years. Thirty years ago the use of vaccines was minimal, nowadays our pets are subjected to a battery of vaccines before they're a few months old. How any animal's system is expected to cope with so many vaccines in such a short time is questionable, and is especially questionable in young kittens and puppies whose immune systems are underdeveloped.

As pet owners we need to ask if routine vaccination is really necessary, consider whether the risks outweigh the benefits, and give thought to the alternatives. We cannot ignore the increasing evidence that vaccinations are linked to many serious and chronic health problems in dogs and cats, as well as people.

The links between your pet having been vaccinated and subsequent health problems aren't always obvious. Adverse reactions don't always happen immediately, they can take weeks, months or even years to show up. Dogs and 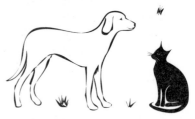 cats are increasingly suffering from degenerative diseases, and at earlier and earlier ages, such as liver failure, kidney failure, thyroid disease, degenerative arthritis, severe skin disorders, digestive disorders, allergies, cancer and other immune deficiency diseases.

'The more vaccines we've developed, the more diseases we've seen.'

Martin Goldstein, DVM

A better alternative?

Homoeopathy offers a harmless alternative to conventional vaccinations in the form of nosodes (preparations of potentised disease products). These can be used as a preventative, instead of vaccines, to protect your pet against specific diseases, such as distemper, parvo virus, feline leukaemia and other diseases that pets are currently vaccinated against. One of the great appeals of using homoeopathic nosodes is that they don't have adverse side effects. Homoeopathic nosodes stimulate the natural defenses of the body to deal with infection when it occurs. They introduce the immune system to harmless profiles of the bacterial/viral protein necessary if it is to defend the body efficiently. They are given by mouth, not by injection. (See Chapter 14 for an explanation of what homoeopathy is and how it works.)

Using homoeopathic preventative treatment

If you decide to use homoeopathic alternatives then get in touch with a homoeopathic vet in your area and seek their advice. Always use homoeopathic nosodes under veterinary guidance (see Chapter 14 for details).

Will my pet be accepted in a kennel or cattery if it hasn't been vaccinated?

There are increasingly more kennel and cattery owners willing to accept proof of homoeopathic protection against disease. To find one in your area contact Canine Health Concern (UK) – see below for details.

The best approach I feel is to keep an open mind, endeavour to become better informed about both sides of the debate, then decide for yourself what you feel is best for your pet. However, the greatest defense against disease is health, and this begins with a good diet and a healthy immune system. It's interesting to note that on his deathbed, the famous microbiologist, Louis Pasteur, turned around his long-held belief that illness was *caused by germs*. His last words were 'seed is nothing, soil is everything'. This is the very foundation of holistic medicine – health is the best protection against disease. A healthy body has an incredible capacity to protect itself against all sorts of invaders.

Ultimately, the question of whether to use homoeopathic alternatives, or conventional vaccines, or neither, is yours; however, the more information you gather on the subject the better able you'll be to make the decision that feels right for you and your pet. (See also Chapters 4 and 5 for diet and supplements, and Chapter 17 for Immune system and infectious diseases.)

Useful information
UK
Canine Health Concern
PO Box 1, Longnor, Derbyshire SK17 OJD
Tel: 07071 226482
Email: K9health@aol.com
Internet: http://members.aol.com/k9health/wwwk9h/index.htm
(Charitable organisation dedicated to better health for dogs and cats providing owners with information on vaccinations, diet, and alternative health care. Quarterly newsletters, seminars and workshops.)

Homoeopathic vets
See Chapter 14 for details.

Suppliers of homoeopathic nosodes for dogs and cats
See Chapter 14 for details.

Further Reading
Vaccination & Immunisation: Dangers, Delusions and Alternatives, Leon Chaitow; The C.W. Daniel Company Ltd, 1987
What Vets Don't Tell You About Vaccines, Catherine O'Driscoll
(Evidence-based book detailing why annual vaccinations are neither necessary, nor safe. Essential reading for any pet owner concerned about conventional vaccinations. Available from Canine Health Concern – see above.)

CHAPTER SEVEN

Acupuncture

AT-A-GLANCE GUIDE

What is it? Acupuncture involves inserting hair-thin needles into the animal's body in an effort to stimulate energy flow and bring about self-healing.

What can it help? Most conditions, physical or behavioural, will respond to treatment.

Can you do it yourself? No. Acupuncture should only be practised by a qualified veterinary acupuncturist.

Average cost per treatment? In line with standard veterinary fees, depending on the length of the consultation.

Does it hurt? No.

Acupuncture is a form of traditional Chinese medicine that has been used in China for over 5,000 years. We know that it has been used on animals for about the same amount of time from the discovery of ancient records and clay models of horses with acupuncture points marked on them.

These days, in China, student vets study acupuncture and Chinese herbs as part of their course.

Acupuncture provides maximum health benefits without the dangerous side effects associated with many modern drugs and surgery.

What is acupuncture?

Acupuncture is based on the belief that health is determined by having a balanced flow of 'chi' (vital life essence) throughout the body. In the West we tend to refer to chi as life-force. An imbalance of chi leads to illness, and so by correcting and rebalancing the flow of chi the body is restored to health. It is a complete system of healing and combines a traditional Chinese diagnosis with treatment using special needles.

The actual treatment involves putting hair-thin needles into specific points along the body in order to stimulate energy flow. These points lie just beneath the surface of the skin and run along energy channels, called meridians, within the body. It is by stimulating the energy flow at these specific points that acupuncture aims to treat disease.

The meridians are named after the organs and systems that they have the most effect on, for example, the heart meridian or the kidney meridian. Often a pain at a specific point along a meridian line may indicate that there is a problem with the associated organ, rather than with the place the pain seems to be coming from.

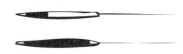

The meridians are not something we can see, in the sense that an anatomist would not tell you there are energy channels in the body. However, the Chinese certainly believe they exist. They believe that the chi flows along these meridians and gets distributed around the whole body. Chi provides the basic vitality for the body's organs and tissues and promotes good health by maintaining body harmony.

What disease does, or the result of the disease processes does, is to interfere with the flow of chi. Acupuncture can influence the energy flow and normalise it, returning the body to a healthy, balanced state where it can ultimately heal itself.

'The principles of acupuncture don't sit easily on conventional Western shoulders because you have the idea of "life-forces" and "lines of energy" which run through the body. Funnily enough,

Western medicine has found that an awful lot of these energy lines are allied to nerve pathways.

Alasdair MacFarlane Govan, BVMS, MRCVS

Do animals enjoy acupuncture?

Acupuncture does not hurt and most vets report that dogs and cats do not seem to mind it and often fall asleep during their treatment. The ones that do not like it are usually animals that do not like being handled anyway. Remember, animals do not have the same psychological fear of needles as some humans do! If the animal is at all nervous, there is an acupuncture point that can be used to calm them before beginning treatment.

Using acupuncture on animals

Acupuncture works in exactly the same way with animals as it does with people except the method of diagnosis is slightly different. An acupuncturist working with people will often ask detailed questions as part of their diagnosis – which you obviously cannot do with pets! However, to use acupuncture fully with animals you still have to make what is called a 'traditional Chinese diagnosis'.

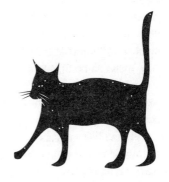

This involves looking at various different aspects of the animal. This could be looking at the coating on the tongue, feeling the animal's pulse, looking at its general condition and observing its behaviour. They may also ask you about your pet's sleeping and eating habits, digestion, urine and so on.

Many vets will also look to see whether it is more of a 'yang' animal or a 'yin' animal. The yang animal is an extrovert, bouncy type of animal, whereas a yin animal is a more quiet type. The Chinese believe that good health depends on the proper balance between yin and yang – two opposing forces, or opposite poles of energy – and an imbalance can result in ill health.

During the diagnosis they will be looking at all of these characteristics to work out what the 'normal' energy is of the body. Taking the pulse gives an idea of the yin-yang element as well as giving an idea of the 'character' of the energy and the strength of the flow. Generally, with veterinary acupuncture, you can expect quite a lot of owner participation, more so perhaps than with orthodox veterinary treatment.

Some vets will not have the time to use acupuncture in a truly holistic way, and use what is called recipe acupuncture. This is where certain points are known to be good for certain symptoms and conditions and does not rely on first making a traditional Chinese diagnosis. However, to use acupuncture to its full healing capacity you really have to make a complete Chinese diagnosis and follow the principles of holistic treatment and treat the whole being, not just the disease symptoms.

Many veterinary acupuncturists will also make an orthodox diagnosis since there are benefits from both Western and Chinese diagnoses, and in some cases it may be best to combine modern drugs with acupuncture.

The acupuncture points in dogs and cats

There are hundreds and hundreds of acupuncture points all over dogs and cats but only about 30 points are commonly used, and not all of these would be used in the same session. More usually a vet works on five or fewer points at a time.

Animals can be treated either standing up or lying down, depending on the vet's preference and which points are being used. Often animals feel quite sleepy during their treatment. The needles may be left in for up to half an hour, but as with all complementary treatments there are no hard and fast rules about how long a session might take. It depends on the animal and what is happening with the energy. Every animal will respond differently.

Why choose acupuncture for my pet?

For a start, you are not giving your pet anything that is going to give it nasty side effects like some drugs can – especially if your pet is going to be on the drugs long term. For example, chronic, painful arthritis can mean that they are on steroid drugs for a number of years. In the end these can be harmful, usually to the liver and kidneys. Acupuncture does not have adverse side effects and treats the body as a whole. Many animals also get a feeling of well-being from the acupuncture that they do not necessarily get from drugs. Acupuncture is an holistic treatment in the sense that although you might have taken your animal in with a particular problem, there might be other underlying things that will also benefit from the acupuncture.

Animals can also greatly benefit from acupuncture when they are ready to die. It has been found that death is more peaceful and occurs with less suffering if the animal has acupuncture treatment.

What can be treated with acupuncture?

Acupuncture is very effective in certain cases and less so in others. Often the cases it is not so effective in are ones where it is used as a last-ditch attempt to cure something.

> 'Unfortunately a lot of people try all aspects of Western medicine first, and go all through that, and then they say "nothing is working, I've heard you can use acupuncture in animals, so let's give it a go". By the time the animal begins treatment it may already be too late to stimulate its own natural healing powers.'
>
> *Alasdair MacFarlane Govan BVMS, MRCVS*

Acupuncture is as much a preventative medicine as it is a potential cure and the sooner an animal is brought for treatment the more likely it is to make a full recovery. With acupuncture the emphasis has always been on prevention.

The emphasis of traditional Chinese medicine is more on prevention than cure and works on the principle that it's better to shut the stable door before the horse has bolted.

Vets who use acupuncture find that the kinds of conditions it can best help include:

- Chronic conditions like arthritis, rheumatism, back problems, gastro-intestinal diseases.
- Musculo-skeletal problems such as hip dysplasia, slipped disc, problems with joints, spinal problems, locomotive problems, some types of paralysis and injuries.
- Pain relief generally and after surgery. Acupuncture has been found to be effective when morphine has not. It stimulates the body's own natural pain-killing chemicals.

- Respiratory problems.
- Skin conditions, allergic dermatitis, hair loss and other types of skin problems.
- Neurological problems such as epilepsy, anxiety and behavioural problems.
- Urinary control and kidney disorders.
- Reproductive disorders. Vets have reported success with treating the heat cycle of bitches, bitches that are continuously getting false pregnancies, or very short heat cycles, balancing hormones.
- Liver problems. It is good for treating the liver.

'We often use it for liver problems because there is not much else you can do anyway, and it really does tend to work very well because there is a very strong energy path from an area of the spine down to the liver.'

Helen Gould BVetMed, MRCVS

- Appetite problems. It is great for encouraging eating, especially with cats, as they can go off their food after surgery.
- Hormonal problems. Almost all the endocrine glands, such as the reproductive organs and the thyroid, can be influenced. Blood sugar control can be normalised in diabetic animals.

For specific ailments, see Chapter 17.

Case histories

'I treated a basset-hound who, when he first came for acupuncture, was walking on his hocks. He had dreadful back legs and his owners had given up on him. He had very slack joints and poor muscular tone and I treated him for about three to four weeks. The dog is actually walking quite well now. It has been to shows and even been placed. That's a success without a doubt.'

'Another lady brought two dogs here and they both had spondylosis of the spine and were slowly but surely losing the power of all their limbs and were heading to be put down. They were sisters and had been referred to me by another vet. And it's quite interesting because the vet she went to had been taking serial

X-rays and could see the spondylosis getting worse and worse. She brought the dogs for acupuncture about once or twice a week for six months and from the time of starting the acupuncture the spondylosis just slowly started to disappear. Those two dogs got better and never needed any more treatment and that was it.'

Alasdair MacFarlane Govan BVMS, MRCVS

How many treatments will my pet need?

It really depends on the individual cat or dog. If you are dealing with a chronic case (a long-term problem) it can take quite a number of treatments before you see any effect. It is important to remember that natural healing methods often take longer to work than drug treatment. Some vets may put a limit on the amount of treatment they will do if there has been no improvement, because it may be that the chance of recovery is slight or that it will take too long. Having said that, most cats and dogs will respond after just one or two treatments.

With acute (short-term) conditions there may be a fairly dramatic response because the energy has not been out of balance for as long and can therefore be corrected more quickly than in chronic situations. With a long-term chronic condition like arthritis, the acupuncture is not really treating the arthritis. What it is doing is removing the pain and letting the animal feel better about everything. This is one of the benefits of acupuncture – it improves quality of life in a situation where the disease process cannot actually be reversed, and it also helps to slow down the disease process. In cases like this you might have to take your pet for a booster dose whenever it needs it, which will vary depending on the animal and the speed of degeneration. Some animals may go a month between appointments, some two months, and it is not unusual for them to go as long as six months.

Can acupuncture be used with other therapies?

Like many other forms of complementary medicine, acupuncture is a complete system of healing that stands on its own and should be respected as such. It is best not to use lots of different therapies and treatments at once. Combining healing with acupuncture, for example, would not be a good idea since they are both working with subtle energies and can interfere with each other, but a more physical treatment, like herbal medicine, would be all right to use at the same time. Acupuncture also complements conventional medicine very well and can be used to enhance its effects.

There is a growing interest in veterinary acupuncture from pet owners who are preferring to use natural treatments and remedies on their pets. Many vets too are feeling that they cannot always adequately treat some conditions with orthodox Western medicine and have added acupuncture to their practice to help them with those conditions.

'I would like to see every veterinary school in this country teach acupuncture as part of the course. It could be integrated with ordinary Western veterinary medicine so that we see people broadening the way that they look at disease, the way they treat disease and actually going for what is best for a particular condition and for a particular animal.'

Helen Gould, BVetMed, MRCVS

A growing understanding and respect for acupuncture, and its place in veterinary medicine, has led to it being increasingly integrated into standard veterinary medicine.

Useful information

Where to find a veterinary acupuncturist
UK
The Association of British Veterinary Acupuncture
Handcross, Haywards Heath, West Sussex RH17 6BD
Tel: 01444 400213
(Send a sae for list of vets who practise acupuncture.)

US
International Veterinary Acupuncture Society
PO Box 271395, Fort Collins, Colorado, 80527
Tel: (970) 266 0666
Email: ivasoffice@aol.com
(IVAS offers courses to vets, and provides a referral service to the public. For information, send a sae.)

Australia

Holistic Animal Therapy Association Of Australia
PO Box 202, Ormond, Victoria 3204
Tel/Fax: (03) 9578 3710

CHAPTER EIGHT

Aromatherapy

AT-A-GLANCE GUIDE

What is it? The use of plant essential oils to treat disease.

What can it help? All sorts of problems, physical, mental and emotional. Also good for first-aid use.

Can you use it yourself? Yes. Essential oils are easy to use and are widely available.

Is it safe? Yes, when used correctly and in the appropriate quantities.

Average cost of treatment? The cost of individual oils varies, some are relatively inexpensive, others are quite expensive. Treatment from a professional aromatherapist will be in keeping with standard consultation fees.

Aromatherapy is the art and science of using plant essential oils to treat both the emotional body and the physical body of animals. It takes into consideration the whole animal, so you are not just treating one specific symptom of illness. The oils work to support the animal's whole being in an effort to rid it of disease.

Like other holistic treatments, aromatherapy puts great emphasis on prevention being better than cure. Essential oils have a positive effect on an animal's whole being – mind, body and spirit – and leave no toxic residue in the way that synthetic drugs do.

What are essential oils?

Essential oils are aromatic essences extracted from a wide variety of trees and plants, such as eucalyptus, pine, geranium, lavender and jasmine. The essential oils are contained in tiny glands in the plants and have potent therapeutic properties. They could even be described as the very 'spirit' or 'soul' of a plant.

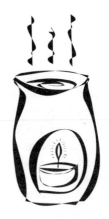

How do they work?

Exactly how essential oils work is something of a mystery, but we know they have active medicinal properties. They seem to work energetically, like the flower essences, and can positively influence an animal's vital force. The energy of the oils interacts with the energy of the animal to produce a healing effect. When an animal's vital force becomes weakened or impaired in some way, then disease follows. You get outward signs that something is wrong, such as a heart condition or a behavioural problem. The root cause of the illness may be physical, emotional, or mental and by rebalancing the vital force, the body is brought back into harmony and health. When you treat an animal with an essential oil, the healing properties are drawn to whichever part of the body is out of balance and in need of healing. By increasing the animal's vital force, its own powers of self-healing are stimulated. Essential oils have a fast-acting therapeutic action on the body and some, like lavender, are adaptogenic, which means they are able to adapt to what the body needs at the time.

Essential oils work to support every aspect of an animal.

The healing properties of essential oils

Not all oils have the same properties, but in general essential oils are antiseptic and detoxifying and help to strengthen the immune system and regulate metabolism. They all contain active chemical constituents, and in many cases modern medicine has taken the individual chemical constituents from the oils and made them into a patented product. For example, thymol, which is used for treating throat and mouth conditions, is extracted from thyme. Thymol is a patented product using one small part of the oil.

> 'In taking a small part of that oil away and making it into a product in its own right, you lose a lot of the synergistic process of that oil, which is all the parts working together to form the cure. So to go back to the concept of holism, looking at the whole animal, I think you need to use the whole product to get an effective cure.'
>
> *Sarah Fisher, aromatherapist*

Essential oils have powerful antiseptic, anti-viral, anti-bacterial and anti-fungal properties. They are detoxifying and revitalising, anti-inflammatory, pain-relieving, relaxing, soothing, and anti-depressant. They can regulate the nervous system and the hormonal system and have a diuretic effect on the body. They can also be used to heal injuries and repel insects.

Because of these wide-ranging curative properties, essential oils can be used to treat a variety of conditions and are especially effective in boosting the immune system, increasing resistance to disease and fighting infection.

Plant essential oils are usually extracted by a process of distillation to capture the healing essence. Plant essential oils are very concentrated which makes them extremely potent even in tiny amounts.

Using aromatherapy with animals

Aromatherapy could be described as a 'branch' of herbal medicine, but, unlike herbs, it is only in the past few decades that aromatherapy has been used on animals – and only very recently has it become a popular treatment, particularly for dogs, cats and horses.

Most animals love aromatherapy, but if this is not the case, the treatment should not be used.

How to use essential oils

Essential oils can be used in a variety of ways, the most common being massage and inhalation.

Baths This is a useful way of using essential oils to combat fleas and other external parasites, and to sooth and heal skin problems. Add a few drops of your chosen oil to water and bathe your pet.

Compresses A compress of essential oils and water helps to relieve bruising, muscle pain and skin problems. Add 3 or 4 drops of essential oil to a bowl of warm water. Soak a piece of cotton in the water, put it over the area to be treated and leave the compress in place for up an hour at a time.

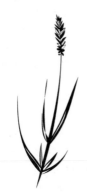

Inhalation Essential oils can be absorbed by inhalation using burners, diffusers or vaporisers which make the essential oils airborne. This is a good way to treat cats, since they are often sensitive to having oils massaged into their skin. Treatment by inhalation is ideal for treating all kinds of respiratory problems and is great for disinfecting places where several animals are kept in a small area, such as kennels and catteries. With infections, like kennel cough and feline flu, using oils in a diffuser is really appropriate because you minimise the spread of that disease to other animals.

A diffuser has an electrical motor that pumps a fine spray of essential oils into the air. The oils can be used undiluted. Diffusers do not heat the oils which makes this method the most attractive. Burners heat the essential oils by a candle or you can use a burner ring placed on top of a warm light bulb. When using burners, dilute the essential oil with water. A vaporiser has an electrical heater and the oils can be used undiluted.

Treatment by inhalation should be done twice a day for a week.

Massage Diluted oils can be gently massaged into an animal's skin where they are very quickly absorbed. Most pets enjoy being touched and find massage relaxing and soothing. Massage is also toning and harmonising and is a good form of treatment for pets that need calming. Touch is very therapeutic and most pets love it. Add 1 or 2 drops of your chosen oil to a tablespoon of almond oil or vegetable oil and lightly massage into the skin for approximately five minutes. For most complaints and conditions you can do this twice a day for a week.

Be careful about using aromatherapy on the skin of cats because they can be hypersensitive which is why a lot of cats have problems with flea collars and flea powders. When you are working with cats, it is best to use the essential oils in a burner, diffuser or vaporiser so that the cat is inhaling the aroma and getting the healing benefits that way.

Neat Lavender and tea tree oils can sometimes be used neat (undiluted) on burns, cuts, grazes, bites and stings.

Taken internally Internal use of aromatherapy is fairly controversial and is practised much more in France than it is elsewhere. Do not give your pet oils to eat unless you are experienced in using essential oils and know exactly what effect you are hoping to achieve. Any internal use of essential oils should be under the guidance of your vet or an experienced aromatherapist. This is because essential oils are very concentrated and it is easy to give an overdose and actually harm your pet. Having said that, taking essential oils internally can be most beneficial for digestive problems, internal parasites and other things. You can mix the essential oils with wheat-germ oil which is high in vitamin E and just add it to their food – but always be mindful of the potency of essential oils.

Dosage
Essential oils are very potent and should always be diluted when used directly on the skin or taken internally. Add 2 or 3 drops of essential oil to 2 teaspoons of a base oil such as almond oil or vegetable oil. You can mix different essential oils and use up to 3 in the same blend.

What can aromatherapy help?
- Digestive problems, allergies.
- Emotional problems, nervousness, stress, anxiety.
- Skin complaints, parasites.
- Respiratory problems.
- Car sickness.
- Arthritis, rheumatism, sprains and strains.
- Viral complaints such as kennel cough and feline flu.
- Infections.

For specific ailments, see Chapter 17.

First-aid use

Also see Chapter 16. Aromatherapy is great for first-aid use. For example, you can use tea tree and lavender or any of the antiseptic oils in a dilution for cuts, grazes and burns. In cases of shock, lavender is a really good calmative. You can massage lavender into their ears – there is a 'shock point' at the tip of the ear which means you can combine the effect of the essential oil with the calming effect of massaging the ears.

Using essential oils yourself

Although each animal is an individual and should be treated holistically, some oils are known to work well for particular conditions (see Chapter 17).

Is it safe?

Aromatherapy oils are very concentrated and need to be used with care. They are safe if you are aware of the properties of the oils and use them in the correct dilutions. They are nearly always used in a diluted form to prevent overdosing and irritation. Some of the essential oils are harmful during pregnancy, and ones to avoid include basil, rosemary, thyme, sage, clary sage and juniper.

The fact that they are natural does not make them safe. You can overdose with essential oils and the reactions can be severe. For example, if you are using rosemary on a dog that has suffered from epilepsy it can provoke an epileptic fit. Some of the citrus oils that are used to keep bugs away are photo-sensitising for animals and can cause sunburn and irritation.

Always keep the oils away from an animal's eyes. If you have an allergic pet, then do a patch test on a healthy part of their body using a diluted oil and wait for at least half an hour to see if there is any adverse reaction.

Always follow professional advice unless you have a good understanding of the individual oils and what they can do because without meaning to you could overdose the animal and potentially cause more problems than you are trying to cure.

> 'I do think there is definitely a place for using aromatherapy on animals but it needs to be reasonably well researched and pet owners need to know what they are doing before they just run to the chemist to get the oils and administer them to their pet.'
>
> *Sarah Fisher, aromatherapist*

Consulting an aromatherapist

For more complicated or serious cases always seek the advice of your vet or ask them to refer you to a qualified aromatherapist. If your vet is not open to holistic treatment find one that is. Usually a homoeopathic vet will be a lot more supportive of other methods of natural healing. Most qualified aromatherapists belong to a governing body. Therefore you can contact one of these and ask for a list of members who work with animals in your area. (See 'Where to find an aromatherapist' for contact addresses and telephone numbers.)

During a consultation the practitioner will take a full case history of your pet and ask about sleeping and eating habits etc to get a 'complete picture' of the disease process in that particular animal. They may also ask you to continue the treatment at home between appointments, using a diffuser or by giving your pet a massage with the appropriate essential oils.

Cost of treatment

Treatment from an aromatherapist is usually in keeping with homoeopathic vets and other natural therapists.

Response to treatment

The effects can be immediate and long-lasting, but how long treatment takes is a bit like asking 'how long is a piece of string?' Every animal is different and much depends on its age, general health and how long the condition has been around. A few days may effect a cure, and a period of three to six weeks is usually long enough to restore balance to the animal's system. Remember that a healthy lifestyle and a natural, preservative-free diet will enhance the healing potential of aromatherapy.

Case histories

'I treated a dog that had a lot of emotional issues and used frankincense with a little bit of lavender for a massage rub into her tummy. She had a lot of fear problems, like a fear of letting go of old patterns of behaviour. She liked the smell of the two oils and frankincense and lavender were the oils that she was most drawn to. It is sometimes a case of watching the animal and letting them pick what they want. Frankincense is really good for dogs who have had abuse problems because it helps them to let go of the past.'

'A cat that I treated had feline leukaemia and had been damaged as a result. Using very weak dilutions, I used 1 drop of frankincense and 1 drop of jasmine to 10mls of vegetable oil and rubbed that on his chest. I asked the owner to continue the treatment at home and to be really careful about not rubbing it right into the skin. I applied it once and said see how it goes over three days. The owner phoned to say she had done it once more and he never sneezed again. Other cats with feline flu could take longer, it depends on how long the illness has been there and what other weaknesses there are, but normally you would get to see an improvement within a couple of days.'

Sarah Fisher, aromatherapist

Is aromatherapy compatible with other treatments?

It is compatible with most other natural therapies and orthodox treatment. It could work against homoeopathy though, and most homoeopaths and aromatherapists will agree between them not to use the two together, because they can cancel each other out. It is probably best not to mix aromatherapy and homoeopathy just to allow each treatment to have its maximum benefit.

Aromatherapy medicine chest for cats and dogs

Eucalyptus Eucalyptus is antiseptic, anti-viral and decongestant. It is a good essential oil if you are dealing with bacterial or viral infections and can be used in a burner or diffuser in the animal's room or in a cattery or kennel. Eucalyptus eases respiratory difficulties. Used with massage it helps ease rheumatism and arthritis. Eucalyptus essential oil is extracted from the leaves and mature branches of the eucalyptus tree.
Cost: Inexpensive

Geranium Geranium is soothing, refreshing and relaxing. Geranium soothes skin irritations, helps to heal burns and minor abrasions. The essential oil is extracted from the whole plant, before it flowers.
Cost: Inexpensive

Lavender Lavender is one of the most useful essential oils and is a must for any first-aid kit. It is good for bacterial and viral problems, it is soothing and helps to heal sore, inflamed areas. Lavender acts as a flea

deterrent, and soothes burns. It is calming and sedative. It is extracted from lavender pods.
Cost: Inexpensive

Marjoram Marjoram is very good at killing airborne bacteria and has strong antibiotic properties. It helps to combat anxiety and stress. Used in massage to treat strained muscles and aching limbs. The essential oil is extracted from the flowering tops and leaves of the herb.
Cost: Fairly expensive

Melissa Melissa is very good for when a pet has died or has had to be put down. Burning melissa oil at these times can help the other animals in the household come to terms with the death. Melissa is also good for treating nervous conditions and stress.
Cost: Expensive

Peppermint Peppermint oil is a good digestive tonic and has anti-spasmodic properties making it useful for colic and other digestive complaints. You can use it on an animal's bedding to keep fleas away by spraying their bed with a solution of peppermint oil, vodka (to dilute the essential oil) and water. Do not put undiluted peppermint oil straight onto their bed because it will go rancid. Peppermint is very cooling and refreshing which makes it particularly good to use in summer on their beds. This is also the time when fleas are at their most prolific. The oil comes from the leaves of the plant.
Cost: Inexpensive

Tea tree is another of the most useful oils and, like lavender, is a must for any first-aid kit. It boosts the immune system and is well-known for

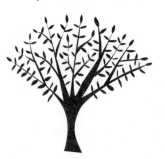 its antiseptic, anti-bacterial, anti-fungal and anti-viral properties. Tea tree is also very good for using as a wash. If you have had a sick animal, you can cleanse the area with tea tree so that other animals do not get the sickness as well. It is good for dandruff and skin disorders including burns, insect bites and warts. The

essential oil is distilled from the leaves and twigs of this common Australian tree.

Cost: Inexpensive

Buying the oils

Many essential oils on the market are not 'pure' essential oil but are blended or synthetic. Even some of those that claim to be 'pure essential oil' may be pure oils which have been mixed with another cheaper oil. For example, a good rose oil should cost over £200 for about 1–2 mls! However, most of the commonly used essential oils are inexpensive. If you do not use pure oils you cannot expect to get a curative result. Synthetic copies simply do not work. Always buy essential oils from reputable sources who specialise in aromatherapy oils for practitioners (see Where to buy essential oils at the end of the chapter).

Storing the oils

Stored correctly, essential oils should last for a few years. Because they are sensitive to heat, light, plastic and air, they need to be stored with care. Essential oils should be stored in tinted glass bottles and kept away from heat and strong sunlight.

Useful information

Where to buy essential oils and aromatherapy products for pets
UK
New Seasons
The Old Post Office, Lockinge, Oxon OX12 8PA
Tel: 01235 821110
Fax: 01235 834294
E-mail: abreaks375@aol.com
Internet: www.newseasons.co.uk
(Stock a range of ready-made aromatherapy products for dogs and cats, such as ear drops, bedding spray, skin creams and shampoo.)

Essentially Oils Ltd
8–10 Mount Farm, Junction Road, Churchill, Chipping Norton, Oxon OX7 6NP
Tel: 01608 659544

Fax: 01608 659544
E-mail: sales@essentiallyoils.com
Internet: www.essentiallyoils.com
(Suppliers of pure essential oils, base oils, burners, vaporisers, diffusers, books.)

Faithful Friends
(For details see Chapter Five.)

US

Aromatherapy International
150 Staniford St, Ste 632, Boston, MA 02114
Tel: 1-800-722-4377 or 617 670-1792
Fax: 617 846-0285
Email: eurolink@umich.edu
(Distributes essential oils grown and distilled by Nelly Grosjean, author of *Veterinary Aromatherapy*.)

Woodland Essence
Tel: (315) 845 1515
(Suppliers of massage oils, wound washes, salves and creams.)

Where to find an aromatherapist to treat your pet
UK
ISPA (International Society of Professional Aromatherapists)
82 Ashby Road
Hinckley
Leicestershire LE10 1SN
Tel: 01455 637987

Further reading
Veterinary Aromatherapy by Nelly Grosjean; The C.W. Daniel Company Ltd, 1994
Tea Tree Oil, A Medicine Kit in a Bottle by Susan Drury; The C.W. Daniel Company Ltd, 1991

CHAPTER NINE

Biochemical tissue salts

AT-A-GLANCE GUIDE

What are they? Tiny sugar-milk tablets containing potentised mineral salts.

What can they help? Many physical and behavioural problems.

Can you do it yourself? Yes, they are perfectly safe and there is no danger of overdosing.

Cost? The tissue salts are relatively inexpensive.

Biochemical tissue salts are potentised preparations of 12 of the most common mineral salts found in the body. They were first developed by a Dr Wilhelm Schuessler, who believed that many diseases were caused by a lack of one or more of these 12 vital mineral salts. For example, a lack of calcium phosphate would lead to teeth problems, and a deficiency of magnesium phosphate would affect the nerves and muscles.

The use of tissue salts is really a branch of homoeopathy. While homoeopathy cures 'like with like', tissue salts treat disease by correcting mineral imbalances inside the body's cells which helps to restore health. Tissue salts are made only from mineral sources, whereas homoeopathic remedies are made from animal, mineral and vegetable sources. (It may be helpful to read Chapter 14 as well, which gives a fuller understanding of how homoeopathy works and the thinking behind it.)

Using tissue salts with animals

Tissue salts have been used successfully on animals for over 100 years. Animals often respond very quickly and there is no danger of nasty side effects.

Animals are instinctive about their health and will naturally try to restore imbalances and deficiencies of important nutrients. This is why they sometimes have peculiar appetites for surprising foods. Research shows that some ailments in animals are directly linked to mineral and trace-element deficiencies.

How do tissue salts work?

The potentised mineral salt takes on healing properties over and above that of the material substance from which it was made. It is like a supercharged version of the original substance – this is in essence the principle of how tissue salts work. They restore the healthy functioning of the cells by stimulating the body's own powers of recovery.

What can they help?

- Digestive problems.
- First-aid cases, such as burns and wounds.
- Behavioural problems, anxiety.
- Skin and coat problems.
- Chronic conditions like rheumatism and arthritis.

For specific ailments and first-aid use, see Chapters 16 and 17.

Treating your pet at home

The key to successful treatment is to match the symptoms to the remedy. Unlike homoeopathy, which builds a whole picture of the disease, the tissue salts are based on the theory that a specific symptom indicates that a specific tissue salt is needed.

Tissue salts are easy to use and there are only 12 basic remedies to choose from.

Giving tissue salts to your pet

The remedies need to be given away from meal times and can be put straight into your cat's or dog's mouth. Because they are soft, they dissolve almost immediately so there is little chance of your pet spitting it out again!

Tissue salts can also be used externally for cuts and wounds. For example iron phosphate tablets can be crushed and rubbed into the affected part (after it has been cleaned). Alternatively, you can dissolve the tablets in sterilised water and make a paste to rub straight onto the skin.

The 12 mineral salts

Calcium fluoride (calc. flour.) Maintains the elasticity of tissues, improves the strength of the heart muscle. Good for arthritis. Strengthens teeth.

Calcium phosphate (calc. phos.) Constituent of bones and teeth. Helpful in cases of bone-healing, indigestion, itching skin.

Calcium sulphate (calc. sulph.) Blood constituent. Good for skin problems, suppurating burns and wounds.

Iron phosphate (ferr. phos.) Minor respiratory disorders, blood-stream oxygenation. Good in cases of inflammation, rheumatism, first stages of fever, wounds, sprains and strains.

Potassium chloride (kali. mur.) Minor respiratory disorders. Cold symptoms, second stages of inflammation, rheumatism and swelling, warts, burns, cystitis, constipation.

Potassium phosphate (kali. phos.) Soothes the nerves. Useful for irritability, anxiety, stress, cystitis, itching skin, bad breath, travel sickness.

Potassium sulphate (kali. sulph.) Maintains a healthy skin and coat. Good for hair loss, eczema, and dandruff.

Magnesium phosphate (mag. phos.) Soft-tissue salt. Good for cramp, colic, cystitis, flatulence. A nerve tonic.

Sodium chloride (nat. mur.) Important for fluid balance. Helpful in cases of watery discharges eg diarrhoea, runny nose. Also good for dandruff, eczema and infertility. Can be applied topically to bites and stings.

Sodium phosphate (nat. phos.) Acid neutraliser. Good for digestive problems.

Sodium sulphate (nat. sulph.) Balances fluids in the body. Used for queasiness, digestive upsets, vomiting, rheumatism.

Silicon dioxide (silica) Skin and coat conditioner. Good for hair loss. General cleanser.

You can also use ready-made combination remedies of two or more tissue salts; for example, combination M for nervousness, anxiety and stress contains calc. phos., kali. phos. and ferr. phos.

Dosage

Like homoeopathic remedies, the tissue salts are tiny sugar-milk tablets which contain the potentised mineral salt. The dosage is the same for dogs and cats and there is no danger of overdosing. Any excess will be eliminated by the body and, since they are harmless, if you prescribe the wrong remedy it will not have any adverse effects. However, like all natural remedies, it is always best to use them in the recommended dose.

Acute, short-term problems: 2 to 4 tablets 3 times a day. In severe cases, 2 to 4 tablets can be given every half hour until the symptoms lessen. If there is no change after a couple of weeks, stop giving the remedy.

Chronic, long-term conditions may need to be treated for a number of weeks. Give 2 tablets, twice a day.

Always consult your vet if your pet's condition is serious.

How quickly do they work?

With acute, short-term conditions your pet may improve within a matter of hours, especially if the tablets are being given every half an hour or so. It can take much longer to notice improvements in long-term conditions, and it can be as much as six months in some cases. A lot depends on the animal's age and breed as well but, in general, the longer a condition has been around, the longer it will take to heal. Do not expect an instant cure; mineral salts, like other natural forms of treatment, work by gradually and gently restoring the body to health and harmony.

Storage

The tablets will keep for about three years if stored in a cool, dry place away from strong light.

Can they be used with other treatments and remedies?

The biochemical tissue salts complement other treatments and therapies well.

Useful information

Where to buy biochemical tissue salts

These are widely available from health-food shops and pharmacies and are made by New Era.

CHAPTER TEN

Chiropractic

AT-A-GLANCE GUIDE

What is it? Gentle manipulation of the spine and skeletal system using only the hands.

What can it help? All kinds of musculo-skeletal problems.

Average cost of treatment? Variable, but usually in keeping with standard veterinary fees.

Can you do it yourself at home? No. Treatment by professionally trained chiropractors only.

Is it safe? Yes. In trained hands.

Chiropractic is a hands-on treatment that aligns and balances an animal's musculo-skeletal system. Much of the treatment concentrates on the spine and its effect on the animal's central nervous system. Just like us, dogs and cats get musculo-skeletal problems, affecting the back, neck, limbs, spine and pelvis, and so they too can be helped by chiropractic.

Like osteopathy, chiropractic probably has its roots in the hands of the old bonesetters until it became an established form of treatment in the 1890s. Nowadays there are several branches of the original chiropractic methods, including McTimoney chiropractic which was developed in 1950 by John McTimoney. It was he who first adapted chiropractic techniques to suit animals, and since then many chiropractors have turned their attention to treating animals.

Chiropractic is known for its gentleness and simplicity which animals accept quite readily. It is a non-invasive treatment and is quite safe in experienced hands. Chiropractic takes account of the animal's whole body and the deeper effects that structural problems can have on internal organs and systems.

How does it work?

Chiropractic aims to align and balance the animal's musculo-skeletal system using light and gentle manipulation techniques. The musculo-skeletal system refers to the whole of the body's structure – the bones, joints, muscles, ligaments and tendons.

Practitioners use only their hands to perform gentle manipulations which cause the animal's own muscles and ligaments to bring the bones back into place. By adjusting any misalignments using swift, but gentle thrusts, the animal's muscles respond and pull the vertebrae back into the correct position naturally.

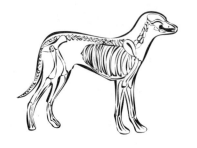

In chiropractic, the spine is seen as a particularly important area of treatment and plays much more than just a structural and supportive role. It also houses and protects the central nervous system. The animal's nerve supply goes right the way down the spine and if a nerve gets pinched or trapped, the electrical impulse cannot be carried down the nerve pathways properly, therefore a major organ, like the heart or the liver, can be adversely affected. Treatment can remove tension and relieve pain. Chiropractic treats the deeper cause of symptoms and is therefore a whole body treatment.

'If you think of the nerve supply as being rather like a hose-pipe, depending on the amount of pressure you put on it, you can either speed up the water or slow it down. The nerve supply is exactly the same, a little bit of pressure can speed up the nerve supply and lead to overactivity of that particular organ or it can cause underactivity if it's pressed a bit harder.'

The Hon Richard Arthur, McTimoney chiropractor

If anything damages the spine or when vertebrae get out of alignment, the rest of the body can be adversely affected. If there is pressure on the nerves they cannot carry out their proper function and this can lead to disharmony and disease. Because of this, when chiropractors work on an animal's body, seemingly unrelated internal symptoms may be cured as a result of the spinal manipulation.

'I won't go ahead and treat an animal for say a kidney problem, but I may well relieve it incidentally while I am treating the spine.'

The Hon Richard Arthur, McTimoney chiropractor

Realigning and rebalancing an animal's body not only restores mobility but also takes any undue pressure off the nerve pathways which are connected to all its major organs and systems.

Chiropractors believe that many disorders originate from a lack of nerve supply and chiropractic enables the cause of this lack of nerve supply to be addressed by correcting any misalignments.

Making a diagnosis

Usually an animal will already have been seen by a vet to get the initial diagnosis before being referred to a chiropractor.

The chiropractor will take account of the vet's diagnosis and discuss this with you, as well as asking you various questions about your pet. Then he will make a physical check of the animal, both by looking at it and feeling it with his hands.

The animal is thoroughly checked in this way for possible misalignments, with particular regard to the spine and the pelvis. Relevant joints and muscles (which may be in spasm) are also checked, as is the animal's full range of movements.

Treating animals

Once the source of the problem has been discovered, the area is treated with gentle but swift manipulations to correct any misalignment and reduce muscle spasm. The practitioner will use only his hands in a gentle and non-intrusive way. The McTimoney chiropractic method is especially famed for its light touch that almost teases the joints and muscles to respond rather than forcing them to respond. This ensures that animals do not suffer any discomfort during treatment.

What can be treated?

• Lameness.
• Uncharacteristic changes in mobility.
• Limb-dragging or irregular limb action.
• Paralysis.
• Joints out of place following a fall or accident.
• Stiffness.
• Trapped nerves, pain.
• Spinal problems.
• General musculo-skeletal problems.

Symptoms of musculo-skeletal problems

• Crying out when getting up.
• Difficulty climbing stairs or climbing in or out of a car.
• Reluctance to exercise.
• Shying away from being stroked along their back.
• Unusual movement for that particular animal.
• Favouring the use of one limb more than another.
• Swelling, stiffness, lameness.
• Irritability.

Dogs

Many breeds are worked hard, especially greyhounds, and this high performance and high expectation can take its toll. Animals like these may often need regular chiropractic treatment as competitive racing places a lot of extra strain on their musculo-skeletal system.

Other breeds, like dachshunds and basset-hounds with long backs can be prone to spinal problems. Simply going up and down an awkward staircase or being overweight can put too much extra pressure on a potentially weak area.

Cats

Cats are not asked to perform in the way that many dogs are, but are just as likely to suffer from musculo-skeletal problems if they have been in a road accident or have fallen from a tree or roof top.

For specific ailments, see Chapter 17.

Preventative treatment

Any animal that is asked to perform beyond the normal life of a pet – like greyhounds, police dogs and sporting dogs – can benefit from preventative treatment. Regular fine-tuning of their structure helps them to perform at their best. The joints and muscles of hard-working animals can also wear out more quickly; regular treatment is therefore a good way of taking care of your animal.

How many treatments?

It is hard to be precise since the effectiveness of treatment depends on many factors, such as the age of the animal, the nature of the problem, how long they have had it. An acute problem (short-term), like a minor accident may take one or two treatments, whereas chronic (long-term) problems may take several treatments. Nature needs time to heal and as long as treatment is having a positive effect, be patient and let it take its natural course.

Is it safe?

Chiropractic is very gentle and has been adapted for use with animals. In trained hands it is perfectly safe and there are no adverse side effects. Your pet will not feel any pain or discomfort since it applies gentle touch and no forceful adjustment is used. Your pet may feel far more discomfort by not being treated!

Case histories

'I've treated a lot of dogs for paralysis, one particular one had fallen and twisted its neck and was completely immobile. I also get a lot that are paralysed in their hind quarters and are totally incontinent.'

The Hon Richard Arthur, McTimoney chiropractor

'Willie, a six-year-old rescue dog had been hit by a car some years earlier and his peculiar, twisted back had always been noted but so far had not caused any problem. One day, he collapsed completely, being unable to walk and in great pain and distress. Chiropractic treatment was sought. Willie was found to have considerable distortion in the pelvis with resultant misalignment in the lower lumbar vertebrae. Within 20 minutes of treatment he was able to get up and run about, to his owners' great joy. He made a complete recovery and went on to live for another 10 years enjoying his rabbiting in the countryside.'

Dana Green, McTimoney chiropractor

Useful information

Where to find a chiropractor

Most chiropractors work closely with vets and have animals referred to them. If you wish to have chiropractic treatment for your pet then talk to your vet and get their co-operation. Most vets are happy to refer an animal to a qualified and experienced practitioner. If your vet does not know of a chiropractor locally you can contact one of the chiropractic associations listed below. They will send you a directory of animal practitioners who are registered and licensed.

UK

McTimoney Chiropractic Association
21 High Street, Eynsham, Oxford OX8 1HE
Tel: 01865 880974
Fax: 01865 880975
(They supply a list of qualified practitioners with additional training in the treatment of animals. They also offer training in McTimoney chiropractic for animals to vets, osteopaths and chiropractors.)

The Oxford College of Chiropractic (Animal course)
c/o Sheilagh Hudson, Old Post Office, Cherry St, Stratton-Audley, Oxon OX6 9BA

Australia

Royal Melbourne Institute of Technology (RMIT)
(Dept of Chiropractic has an animal chiropractic course.)
PO Box 71, Bundoora, Melbourne, Victoria 3083

US

American Veterinary Chiropractic Association
PO Box 249, Port Byron, Illinois 61275
Tel: (309) 523 3995
(AVCA runs teaching courses and seminars and offers a referral service to the public.)

Flower essences

Flower essences work primarily on the emotional and mental levels of an animal and can help to restore health and harmony to its whole being. They make a great healing tool to use at home, especially since they are easy to use on pets, are powerful yet harmless, and are relatively cheap!

Animals are sensitive to changes in their environment which, if adverse, can lead to behavioural problems or physical disease. Anyone who is closely involved with animals will know they can experience fear, despondency, loneliness and depression just as we do and can pick up on our fears and frustrations. The human–animal bond is a close one and pets are particularly vulnerable to absorbing their owners' moods and emotions. Flower essences have the power to heal negative emotions and make a powerful addition to your animal's health care.

The history of flower power

Flowers have been used for thousands of years throughout the world as one of many different natural healing traditions. Like herbs, they are one of the earliest forms of medicine. The healing property of flowers is nothing new, it is just that the knowledge of their curative power was temporarily lost, particularly in the Western world where modern medicine took over from natural healing.

In Europe the use of flowers as remedies was 'rediscovered' and brought back into use by a British physician, Dr Edward Bach (1886–1936), who developed 38 different essences. His philosophy was 'A healthy mind ensures a healthy body' having found that once he had treated his patients' psychological state, their physical symptoms often disappeared too.

He enjoyed nature and observed how flowers could influence his mood, each different flower having a specific effect. While developing his remedies he discovered that when he was in a particular state of

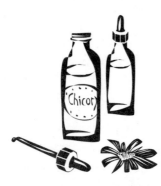

mind or feeling a particular emotion, certain plants and flowers could relieve that emotion. From this he developed his 38 remedies which he believed covered the whole range of human and animal emotions.

Although the most well-known flower essences are the Bach Flower Remedies, based on common British trees and plants like holly, impatiens and oak, there are many others from all over the world including the Hawaiian Tropical Flower Essences, the Australian Bush Flower Essences and the Himalayan Flower Essences.

What are they?

Flower essences are a form of vibrational medicine. They work in a similar way to homoeopathic medicine in the sense that they are both an energetic imprint of the original substance. If you analysed the remedies scientifically you would not find a material amount of the original flower present.

How do they work?

Many forms of natural medicine are based on the belief that illness begins on emotional, mental or spiritual levels before it becomes apparent on the physical. For example, anger can manifest itself as a liver problem, mental rigidity can lead to arthritis, and grief can become cancer. Because of this, by healing the emotional state, the body can be completely cured. As animals are emotional beings, they are just as affected by trauma, grief, loss, or abuse as people are. Because they are so sensitive to subtle energies, the flower essences have a remarkable healing effect on them.

Animals also absorb a lot of stress from their owners. When we are stressed we stroke a cat, or we talk to our dog – and subconsciously they absorb our stress.

'Some people say that they get on much better with their pets than anybody else around! which is why we are so connected to our pets, especially to cats and dogs. The mere fact that they have nice, soft coats that you can stroke calms our nervous system down.'

Clare Harvey, UK's leading authority on flower essences

Flower remedies act as a catalyst which boosts the animal's own powers of self-healing and balances its vital energy.

'I firmly believe that what sets flower essences apart from other forms of remedies is their ability to address physical, mental, emotional and spiritual aspects of the whole being to bring about a complete healing.'

Clare Harvey, UK's leading authority on flower essences

Flower essences work by bringing out positive emotions and getting rid of negative ones.

▼

This is not like the effects of a mood-enhancing drug, which falsely changes an emotional state. Flower remedies work by unlocking inherent positive emotions and bringing them to the surface. For example, if you give an intolerant animal the beech flower remedy this will help to bring about a tolerance of others from within the animal. Hornbeam will help a weak, despondent animal to find a renewed vitality and interest in its daily life.

'The remedies help us to feel ourselves again, at a point where we ceased to be quite ourselves.'

Dr Edward Bach

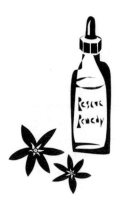

With animals, positive results can happen quickly because they are very direct in their emotions, thoughts and feelings about things and so they can respond very quickly to essences. It is a simple and direct form of medicine for animals and helps them to become healthier and happier.

For an at-a-glance guide to the 38 Bach flower remedies traditionally used for certain emotional states, see page 220.

Rescue remedy is a unique combination of five Bach flower remedies: rock rose for terror; impatiens for impatience; clematis for dreaminess, lack of interest in the present; star of Bethlehem for the after-effects of shock; cherry plum for fear of the mind giving way.

What can be treated with flower remedies?

The most effective use for flower remedies is treating emotional and mental problems. They can reach deep into the animal's being and effect change at a very profound level – therefore all types of behavioural problems can be helped. Although flower essences primarily work on the emotional level, some of the essences also influence the physical body. These include hornbeam for giving strength, crab apple for clear-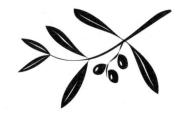

ing out toxins and olive for exhaustion. Some of the flower essences from other parts of the world also have very potent anti-viral and anti-bacterial properties.

Commonly treated problems include:

- Anxiety, fear.
- Bereavement, loss, depression.
- Aggression, jealousy, biting, scratching.
- Hyperactivity, oversexed animals.
- Stress, shock, trauma, accidents, during and after whelping.
- Abuse, neglect.
- Viruses.

For specific ailments and first-aid use, see Chapters 16 and 17.

Treating animals

Flower essences treat animals in a holistic way, treating the whole being, not just the disease symptoms. With flower essences you can tailor-make a mixture of remedies or use just one at a time, depending on what is needed. If you do miss the mark there are no side effects, but it is always better to take your time and choose remedies that will best bring about positive changes.

Remember, when you treat your animals, treat yourself at the same time. Animals really do mirror our emotions and that may be the root cause of their illness. By treating both the pet and its owner (and sometimes the whole household!), you usually get a more effective and long-lasting cure. If you have also been through a stressful situation with your animal, like breaking up a dog fight, then you may benefit from taking one or more of the same remedies as your pet.

'You get a speedier healing of an animal if you can treat the owner at the same time. Often people bring me their animal for treatment and as their pet starts to get better they say, "Well I will come along and have some too." That often happens, especially if there is a very close bond then it is actually quite important to treat both the animal and the owner. Usually when the owner does come I find I am using some of the same remedies on them as I was on their pet.'
Clare Harvey, UK's leading authority on flower essences

Case histories

'I usually recommend rescue remedy in situations involving the collapse of any young animal. It's a means of buying time. It's an excellent adjunct to any other treatment used for and during an immediate crisis. Try it; don't be concerned with (why or) how it works, since you might deprive yourself of a wonderful healing tool.'

J.G.C. Saxton, BvetMed, MRCVS (taken from Rescue Remedy *by Gregory Vlamis, Thorsons, 1994)*

'A lady approached me for remedies for her two cats. TOC, a three-year-old female who had previously been treated with indifference and impatience by her first owners, was hyperactive and continually jumping on the older cat, Mrs Green, who was frightened by TOC's behaviour. Mrs Green had always let herself be pushed around by other cats, never standing up for herself, and her owner described her as a nervous cat, always holding back from strangers. TOC was given agrimony (for her restlessness), vervain (for her hyperactivity), impatiens (for her agitation, always moving around at breakneck speed), beech (to allow her to be more tolerant of Mrs Green), and finally chicory (to address her 'don't ignore me' behaviour towards the owner). Mrs Green was given larch (to boost her self-confidence), mimulus (to give her courage), and centaury (to allow her to be more assertive in the face of TOC's dominance). After a month, the owner wrote to say that Mrs Green was much bolder and not so nervous and had begun to stick up for herself against TOC. TOC was more tolerant towards Mrs Green and had stopped racing around the house at breakneck speed. She added that she had forgotten to mention that Mrs Green had been suffering from halitosis but does not have it any more and wondered if this could have been improved by the remedies as well!'

Christine Newman, registered Bach flower remedies practitioner

Choosing remedies for your pet

The main difference between animals and humans is that you cannot ask animals how they feel. However, you can observe their behaviour and characteristics and make an educated guess. If you know you have a nervous cat who has also experienced some kind of shock, then you would give it remedies for shock and stress – maybe rescue remedy and aspen. It is a question of getting to know your pet and how they react to things.

It can really help if you put yourself in your pet's skin, so to speak. For example, if an animal has just been in a fight, imagine how you would feel after a fight – perhaps a mixture of shock, fear and generally feeling out of sorts. By doing this you can get a fair idea of what emotions the animal is going through. You might have a dog with a hurt leg who is trying to soldier on as if nothing was wrong – this might indicate an oak temperament where the animal is exhausted but struggles on regardless. Another dog might slink off into a corner and be irritable and snappy, which could indicate the need for willow for resentment.

A cat that is normally aloof by nature may become extra aloof when it is ill, and so you could give it water violet. This would be treating the animal's normal character as well as its specific reaction to the illness. Another cat that is normally aloof may become scared and anxious when ill and so you could give it both water violet and aspen together. When prescribing remedies for animals, its 'normal' temperament needs to be taken into account together with its specific mood. When an animal is ill, its mood will often change. Just like humans, animals may get very drowsy and lethargic and need clematis and wild rose or they may seem unpredictable and snappy and need something like holly.

Can you use several remedies at once?
You can use up to six remedies at the same time – but you need to make sure they complement each other which is why it is important to spend time making a good diagnosis. You cannot do any harm by giving the wrong remedies – an animal's body just gets rid of them and there are no side effects – but it is better if you can be as accurate as possible in order to achieve a complete healing. Note that rescue remedy still counts as one remedy, even though it is already a mixture.

Flower essences provide a gentle, safe system of emotional stress relief.

Can they be used with other remedies and therapies?
You can use flower remedies at the same time as orthodox drug treatment, as they will speed up the healing process and help to clear out the drug side effects.

In general, the flower essences complement all forms of natural medicine very well and can be used either as a total system on their own or as part of a broader therapeutic treatment.

Using flower essences at home

Flower remedies really do lend themselves to home use because they are simple to use and easy to get hold of. There are hundreds of different essences from all over the world that can be used. Start by getting to grips with the Bach range, then explore some of the other flower essences as you become more experienced and more knowledgeable.

Dosage

The dosage is the same for cats and dogs as it is for people, usually 3 or 4 drops in their food or water. Drinking water should be fresh every day, so you need to remember to add more drops each time it is changed. If your pet is not drinking much water, put the drops in their food to ensure they are getting the remedy regularly. When flower essences are given in food or water there is no need to worry about other pets in the house accidentally getting a dose too, they will not have any effect unless they are needing the same remedies – and the effects will be positive!

Another way of giving the remedies to cats and dogs is by putting it on their nose and they will lick it off, alternatively you can put it onto their skin and it gets absorbed straight into their system.

Ideally the essences should be given 3 or 4 times a day. In cases of extreme stress they can be given every 10 to 20 minutes until there is some relief.

Length of treatment

There are no hard and fast rules, since complementary medicine is geared towards each individual animal. Pets with an acute condition, like shock, can be given a remedy every 15 minutes until they begin to calm. At the other end of the scale, when dealing with deeply ingrained emotional problems like the lingering effects of a past trauma, the healing process may take several months and they may only need 3 or 4 drops once a day.

Storing the remedies

It is important to remember that the flower essences are liquid energy and can be influenced by other energies. It is particularly important to keep them away from any electrical appliances like televisions, computers, the mains electricity supply and so on. Also keep them away from direct sunlight and strong smells like essential oils and peppermint. Like most medicines, if you store them in a cool, dry cupboard they should be fine. Correctly stored, flower essences will keep for at least five years.

Flower essences as preventative medicine

Flower essences work very well as preventative medicine because, caught early enough, stresses and strains on the emotional level can be prevented from later coming out as physical disease or behavioural problems. This is why it is good to have a bottle of rescue remedy handy, because whenever your pet experiences a shock or stress you can give some to the animal immediately. An accident or fight can often be the trigger that weakens the body system, and the essences pull the system back together again. It is an invaluable remedy to have on tap as part of your first-aid kit for pets.

> 'I have had animals, one for example, which was in an accident and was obviously unconscious and was given a couple of drops of rescue remedy and was immediately brought round into consciousness. So it works that quickly with them.'
> *Clare Harvey, UK's leading authority on flower essences*

Many vets use rescue remedy as a last resort after standard treatment procedures have failed and have reported remarkable results.
(Taken from *Rescue Remedy* by Gregory Vlamis, Thorsons, 1994)

Using flower essences to help a dying animal

Flower essences can help the end of an animal's life to be much more bearable, whether it dies naturally or has to be put down by a vet. The essences also help owners who are upset and distressed watching a much-loved companion pass away. Flower essences can be used to make the last days more positive; they help to make the situation less traumatic and help you to be more accepting.

Bach flower remedy medicine chest

If you only have one flower essence in your medicine chest then make it the rescue remedy. You might be surprised how often you use it, not just for your pet, but for yourself too! However, if you are wanting to have a wider range of essences, the following is a list of some of the most commonly used Bach flower remedies for dogs and cats.

Dogs

Aspen For the nervous, fearful dog, especially in new circumstances. This dog often has its tail between its legs, and may be a submissive wetter. It can help dogs that have been harshly disciplined in the past.

Chestnut bud Helpful in training situations. Useful in teaching a puppy to make a distinction between right and wrong. For example, the difference between a rawhide bone and your shoes! It helps to break bad habits.

Clematis Dogs will sometimes need clematis when kept indoors in stormy weather or when pining for their owner to come home. It can also be used if they are drowsy, but not really sleepy. It is useful following surgery to help them wake up after an anaesthetic. It may be used in combination with rescue remedy the moment puppies are born to help them wake up and breathe.

Chicory For a dog that follows you around, is constantly underfoot, and becomes extremely upset when left alone. For the jealous or possessive dog. For the affectionate dog who always wants to be in your lap.

Holly For the angry dog who threatens attack, or attacks without provocation. Remember that any personality changes should be checked out with a vet. In addition, holly can be useful in treating aggressive behaviour often due to trauma or abuse in the past. (Use star of Bethlehem as well if there has been past trauma.)

Honeysuckle For the dog whose owner or close companion has died or gone away. (Use it in conjunction with star of Bethlehem, especially if the animal's owner or close animal companion has died.) For the dog that acts withdrawn, subdued or unenthusiastic towards people.

For homesickness while at kennels or if left alone for long periods of time.

Mimulus For a dog with a particular fear of known things such as loud noises, thunderstorms, vacuum cleaners, or small children. When these fears turn to terror, use rock rose or rescue remedy.

Olive For the dog who is totally exhausted from illness, hard work or trauma. This remedy may lend a measure of strength and comfort to seriously ill dogs along with star of Bethlehem for physical or emotional trauma.

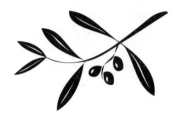

Scleranthus Can be useful in car sickness, used along with the rescue remedy. Also good for seizures.

Vervain For highly strung, hyperactive dogs with a great deal of nervous energy. For those who are hard to stop from jumping up or barking. Where enthusiasm goes with the species, this remedy can help in slowing them down.

Star of Bethlehem For the physically or emotionally traumatised dog, either currently or in the past. Nearly always indicated for dogs that have been in a rescue centre or dog pound. For abused animals.

Water violet Useful for dogs that are aloof, self-reliant, intelligent, and loners. Useful for dogs that were socialised comparatively late in life, and who seem very stand-offish. Often an excellent choice for dogs who have wild ancestry like the husky. It can be used for grieving animals that want solitude.

Rescue remedy Appropriate for any kind of accident, illness, or injury your dog may experience. Can be used at dog shows, on car trips, while boarding, during a long absence, before or after surgery, or whenever a dog seems to be experiencing the effects of extreme stress.

Cats

Aspen For the fearful cat that is always slinking from safe place to safe place, never being quite at ease. Startles easily at any sound, even non-threatening sounds it has heard before.

Beech For picky eaters. For cats that have no tolerance for another animal or certain people. Effective with walnut to assist in keeping the peace between two cats who seem to be fighting. Good for jealous cats when a new person or animal joins the family.

Chicory For the extremely affectionate cat that can be possessive and jealous, always stays near you wanting to be held, petted and fussed over.

Clematis Any time a cat appears stunned or experiences unusual patterns of sleeping beyond the typical catnap. Used in helping to regain consciousness after an accident or operation. Can be used in conjunction with rescue remedy to help newborn kittens wake up and breathe. One drop can be repeated every few minutes.

Honeysuckle For grief or homesickness. For the cat who has lost a person or other animal they have been close to. Star of Bethlehem can be used as well to address this condition. Also helpful along with walnut to help the cat adjusting to a new location.

Hornbeam For fatigue. The strengthening remedy. Can be helpful in assisting runts or to build up any sickly animal.

Larch Especially useful for the low cat in the pecking order, perhaps the runt. For the cat with little or no self-confidence. Self-esteem is an important part of feline well-being and is usually radiated by an emotionally balanced cat.

Mimulus For fear of particular things or circumstances such as thunderstorms, vacuum cleaners, visits by small children. Where fear turns to terror, use rock rose or rescue remedy.

Star of Bethlehem For all trauma, past and present, physical or emotional. For recuperation from surgery, car trips, injury, boarding and other traumas that affect your cat's dignity, freedom, health or security. For cats adopted from shelters.

Vine For the boss cat. One who rules the roost and the household. Vine can make boss cats more tolerant of their companions.

Walnut Very helpful for any sort of changes that a cat may experience, such as new babies or new pets in the house, moving, weaning, or heat cycles. It helps ease adjustment to holidays and changes to the normal routine.

Water violet A constitutional remedy for most cats that helps them keep their instinct for solitude in balance with enjoyable interactions with other animals and people. For aloof, loner animals. Good for grieving or sick animals that want solitude.

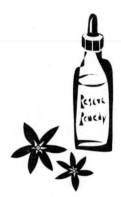

Rescue remedy Appropriate for any kind of accident, illness, or injury your cat may experience. Can be used at cat shows, on car trips, while boarding, during a long absence, before or after surgery, or whenever a cat seems to be experiencing the effects of extreme stress.

Useful information

Where to find a registered Bach flower remedy practitioner
Like most other forms of complementary medicine, many vets are happy to refer you to a qualified practitioner. If your vet does not know of a practitioner who works with animals, then find someone yourself and ask your vet if they will refer your pet.

UK
The Edward Bach Centre
Mount Vernon, Sotwell, Wallingford, Oxon OX10 OPZ
Tel: 01491 834678
Fax: 01491 825022
E-mail: mail@bachcentre.com

Internet: www.bachcentre.com
(The Bach Centre will provide a list of registered practitioners in the UK who work with animals. Also Bach flower essences, general advice, information, education, training, practitioners, newsletters etc.)

Where to buy flower essences
UK
The Edward Bach Centre (see above)

The International Flower Essence Repertoire
The Living Tree, Milland, Near Liphook, Hampshire GU30 7JS
Tel: 01428 741572
Fax: 01428 741679
E-mail: flower@atlas.co.uk
(Stockists of a range of flower essences from around the world – including the Australian Bush Flower remedies, the Healing Herbs of Edward Bach and the Wild Earth Animal Essences.)

Ainsworths Homeopathic Pharmacy
They make their own range of Bach flower remedies.
(For details see Chapter 14.)

Acorn Supplements Ltd
(For details see Chapter 5.)

US
Ellon USA, Inc.
644 Merrick Road, Lynbrook, New York 11563
Tel: (516) 593 2206
Fax: (516) 593 9668
E-mail: rbrody01@interserv.com

CHAPTER TWELVE

Healing

AT-A-GLANCE GUIDE

What is it? Healing uses natural energy to stimulate an animal's own self-healing ability.

What can it help? Almost any condition, physical or behavioural, will benefit from healing.

Can you do it yourself? Yes. There are short courses on animal healing open to vets and non-vets.

Average cost of treatment? Variable, but usually less than standard veterinary fees.

Usually pets enjoy having healing and know instinctively what it is and how it can help them.

Like most animals, dogs and cats are highly sensitive to energy. They seem to 'know' things before we do, and that is why we credit them with having a 'sixth sense'. It is this ability to tune into subtle influences that guides migratory birds across the world and lets animals know when there is a fierce storm brewing. Because healing is an energy medicine, it offers them something natural which they immediately recognize in a way that most humans do not.

Animals have a highly developed sensitivity and they often pick up on our fears and anxieties. This is especially true for domestic pets who soak up any negative emotions around the family home and often become ill or disturbed as a result.

Very often when a pet becomes ill, their owner will be out of sorts as well.

How does it work?

Healing is simply the channelling of energy, or life-force, through the healer into the animal. A healer acts as a link between this energy and the dog or cat, the energy usually being transmitted though their hands – hence the expression 'hands on healing'.

It is a non-intrusive therapy, in the sense that nothing physical penetrates the body and no remedies are given. It is gentle and safe, yet very powerful.

Like other complementary therapies, healing treats the whole being not just the disease symptoms. Without a harmonious balance between the mind, body and spirit, both people and animals eventually become ill. Because healing is such a profound therapy it can reach depths that many other types of medicine cannot.

Healing is one of the oldest forms of medicine in the world and was practised by all the ancient societies and cultures, from the Aborigines in Australia to the South-American Indians.

There are a variety of different healing methods that you may come across including spiritual healing, Reiki, natural healing, and crystal healing, all of which are essentially doing the same thing – using natural energy to restore health and well-being to an animal.

What is this healing energy?

It has many names depending on individual understanding, beliefs and cultures. For example, in the West it is often called the life-force, God force, nature, or divine energy. The Chinese know it as 'chi' and in Indian medicine its called 'prana'. However, the different names are less important than the understanding of what it is and where it comes from. Healers believe that this energy is all around us and within us and comes from one invisible, intelligent source. It is the energy flow in all of life, and what animals are recognizing is that they are a part of it, in the

▼

same way that plants and trees flow with the seasons and follow nature's infinite cycle of creation and decay.

Some people call this energy a love, a deep, unconditional love; animals recognise this deep caring and how it can heal, in the same way that a child recognises that a mother's love can heal many hurts.

Healing animals

By tuning into the life-force the healer can transmit the healing energy to the animal. This helps to balance energy throughout the body; it stimulates the immune system, repairs tissues, revitalises an exhausted animal, calms distress, eases pain and gives an animal a greater sense of well-being.

Animals are very sensitive to healing energy and naturally understand it to the extent that they often offer the parts of them that are affected towards the healer's hands. For example, if there's something wrong with a cat's paw it might offer its paw, or if a dog has a pain in its stomach it might lie on its back and expose its stomach. They work with the healing energy and it almost becomes like a dance where the animal and the healer are working in harmony.

In a way, healing is like jump-starting a car: it gives the animal's whole being a boost of energy and stimulates self-healing.

Which problems can healing help?

Healing can be effective for almost any illness because it is a truly holistic therapy. However, as with any natural treatment, every animal is an individual and will respond in different ways and to different degrees. The types of conditions that healers commonly treat include the following:

- Skin conditions, both long-term and short-term.
- Arthritis, rheumatism, musculo-skeletal problems.
- Cancer (and other 'incurable' conditions).
- Behavioural problems such as nervousness or anxiety.
- Pain relief.
- Digestive problems.
- Respiratory problems.
- Trauma such as past abuse, maltreatment.

Healing can be of real benefit to 'incurable' diseases, and although it may not effect a complete cure, healing can improve the quality of your pet's life. Many people have observed that their animal is much happier and more content even though the illness is still there.

Where behavioural problems are concerned, pets often pick up their owner's anxieties and then display behavioural problems as a result. For example, if their owner is frightened of being left alone or of being in the dark, the pet picks up on these anxieties and starts behaving differently. Whereas the owner might not realise the extent of their own problem, they often see it in their pet and take the animal for healing. An experienced healer will notice what is happening and suggest the owner has healing too.

Behavioural problems may also stem from a trauma, such as a fight with another dog or a frightening experience. Healing is especially useful for animals that have suffered a degree of abuse or neglect in the past. In the same way that you would take a 'rescued' cat or dog to the vet to have a check-up, healing helps pets to settle into a new home much more smoothly.

For specific ailments, see Chapter 17.

Why take your animal to a healer?
Healing is one of the most gentle and natural of therapies and can reach the very soul of an animal. It stimulates an animal's own powers of recovery and does not rely on any medicines or remedies. If you wish to try an alternative or complement to standard veterinary care, then healing offers a powerful treatment. It is especially profound when dealing with behavioural problems, and long-term conditions like eczema and arthritis, which orthodox medicine often cannot help. Healing can improve the quality of life of a dying animal and can help that animal to go more peacefully when it is ready.

Sometimes a condition does not appear to be serious to the untrained eye, so it's vital to get a vet's diagnosis before deciding to seek complementary treatment. As long as the vet has seen your pet then a healer will be happy to see them too.

What to expect in a consultation
Some animals seem to sense the healing energy already in the room when they arrive for treatment and immediately become very still. It

can be astonishing to witness the way that a really frisky animal will suddenly go really still, lie down and become very quiet. Other animals might react in a completely different way, sniffing around the room to identify the energy before settling down.

During the consultation the healer may ask you questions about the nature of your pet's symptoms; for example, what diagnosis has been made, what medication it is on and what recommendations the vet has made so as not to conflict with that advice. The healer may also ask about the animal's bowels, appetite, diet, sleeping and peculiar habits, if any, and offer advice on your pet's diet and recommend vitamin or mineral supplements.

During the actual healing, healers place their hands on or near to the animal and work over its body. How long he spends on each area will depend on how much that part needs, which is really an intuitive feeling on the healer's part. Some animals, especially cats, may not want to be touched at all, so healers place their hands close, without actually touching them. If it is an aggressive animal, again they will heal at a distance. Healing is just as effective this way; however most animals enjoy being touched. Something I often experience when healing cats that won't let you touch them is that when they come for a second treatment it is as if they are a different cat and will let you place your hands anywhere without a fuss! They are recognising the healing and how it can help them.

On average, healing takes about 10 to 20 minutes but it really depends on the animal. A highly frisky dog like a bearded collie may take its healing quickly while on the run, whereas a more relaxed type of dog like a labrador may lie down straight away and not move again until it has had its fill. In both cases the animal will be getting as much healing as it needs at the time. Often they let you know when they have had enough by getting up and wandering off.

Do animals enjoy healing?

Animals seem to enjoy it and usually settle down to receive the healing pretty quickly.

Healing is very soothing for an animal in pain or distress, and even healthy animals can benefit from regular healing to keep them well. I used to give regular healing at an animal sanctuary to a ewe who had a crippled back leg. Every time I began to give her healing some of the other animals, particularly the dogs, would try to nudge in to get a piece of the action! It got to the stage where I had to take the sheep into an enclosed pen so that I could keep all the other animals out while she received her treatment! This was definitely a case where animals were sensing the healing energy and wanting to have some themselves.

How many sessions will my pet need?

This is not something that you can predict since it really depends on how well the animal absorbs the healing and what changes come about. A healer would be unlikely to recommend a specific number of treatments in advance; they are more likely to decide after each appointment whether another one is needed, having assessed how the animal is getting on. Usually, however, you will notice some change after the first healing. A few of the most common things that people report is that their pet seems 'calmer', 'more peaceful', 'more like itself'.

Is healing always about a cure?

Healing is not just about helping an animal to recover from illness or helping it to live well. It is also about helping it to die well. In my own practice I have given healing to several pets with terminal cancer whose vets cannot do any more for them. Usually their owners will bring them for healing to help their pet to be as comfortable as possible for the time they do have left. Others are concerned that their pet dies in a dignified and peaceful way.

A healer will never influence anyone's decision on whether or not to have their pet put down; this decision has to be what the owner feels is right for them and for their animal. It can be a very traumatic experience to watch an animal losing its faculties, as anyone who has witnessed an ill pet will know. If you do decide to have your pet put down, healing can help them to go in peace.

Sometimes it seems as if an animal is hanging on to life when it really should have passed away. In cases like that a healer may explain how you can 'talk' to the animal about it, not necessarily outwardly, but inwardly, and for a lot of people this really does help them to let their pet go. Time and again pets seem to wait for their owners to go off on holiday and then die while they are away. It is as if they are sparing them the experience of coping with their death. So there can be a need for 'talking' to the animal, and for saying inwardly to the animal 'I love you, but I shall let you go to do whatever is right for you.'

Distant healing

Distance healing is a way of giving healing to an animal without the healer actually being present. Healing energy can still be channelled to pets at a distance, whether it's from a few feet away or thousands of miles. This can be a really good way to treat animals who are too ill to get to a healer. It can also be used to begin the healing process until the animal's appointment.

Healing at home

Healing is a wonderful thing and comes naturally to a parent comforting an injured or sick child. In the same way, loving touch and compassion for a sick or dying animal is very healing – and everyone is capable of doing that. However, if you would like to learn more about healing animals there are courses you can go on that will give you an under-standing of animal healing.

Healing as a first-aid/emergency measure

If a healer is present at an accident, a lot of good work can be done immediately. Healing helps to detraumatise the animal, relieve pain and bring it to a more peaceful state, which makes recovery easier.

When an animal has been in an accident it is vitally important it goes to the vet for a check-up even if it looks as if there is nothing wrong. It can have healing afterwards. If there are not any actual injuries, healing can help the animal to recover itself again and reduce the trauma. If there are injuries then it will help to speed up the healing process in the tissues and bones. You could ask your healer if they will come to your home or to send distant healing if you feel the animal is not well enough to travel.

Can healing be used with other therapies?

Like other forms of complementary medicine, healing is a complete treatment on its own. It is therefore best not to use it simultaneously with similar therapies, such as flower remedies, acupuncture and homoeopathy which also work with subtle energy. It does complement the more physical types of treatments, like nutrition, chiropractic, herbal medicine and conventional veterinary treatment and can help to enhance their effects.

Referrals from vets?

Healers try to work in harmony with vets, and more and more vets these days are becoming interested in complementary medicine and are happy to make referrals. Others may practise some form of natural treatment themselves; a lot of vets are taking training in natural medicine in order to incorporate it into their practice because they know of the profound effect it has on animals. Animal healing is no exception to this growth in complementary treatment for pets.

Case histories

'We had a six-month-old puppy here whose owners were told by the vet that nothing more could be done for it and it had to be put to sleep. It was paralysed and couldn't move its legs, and had to be carried in on the first visit. On the second visit it walked in, and on the third it ran in and the owners were saying what difficulty they had restraining it from leaping about! That was lovely.'

'We also had a cat that didn't purr brought to us. It was also always scared and anxious. When it came into the waiting-room it started to purr and that was the first time they had ever heard it purr. And it was just coming into the waiting room. What was happening was that the cat was picking up the caring, the love and the relaxation of the healing energy so it felt able to let go.'

Christy Casley, healer

No list of case histories would be complete without the story of my own dog, Basil. I got him aged one from a rescue centre and as I was driving away with him in the back of the car I heard a faint voice in the distance shouting 'He doesn't like being left alone.' Well, that proved to be an understatement! The first time I left him alone he ate the door frame around the back door in an attempt to get out. The second time I left him in my car for half an hour. When I returned he was in a high state of anxiety and had completely destroyed the inside of the car! Teeth marks on the steering wheel and dashboard, safety belts, car seat, head rests in tatters. (The insurance company covered the repair costs of over £600!) I immediately booked an appointment for him with a local healer and it was as if he became a different dog after just one healing. He has never done anything like that since – he is now nine. The power of healing never ceases to amaze me and time and again I see animals responding in wonderful ways to this ancient art.

Useful information

Where to find an animal healer
Most trained and qualified healers belong to a healing organisation (members are bound by a strict code of conduct in relation to treating animals) and can be contacted through them.

UK
International Self Realization Healing Association
1 Hamlyn Road, Glastonbury, Somerset BA6 8HS
Tel: 01458 831353
Fax: 01458 835148
Email: isrha@btinternet.com
(ISRHA supplies a list of its animal healer members.)

National Federation of Spiritual Healers
Old Manor Farm Studio, Church Street, Sunbury-on-Thames, Middlesex TW16 6RG
Tel: 01932 783164
Email: office@nfsh.org.uk
(The NFSH supplies a list of its animal healer members.)

Foundation for Animal Healing
Charles Siddle
34 Jacks Hill Park, Graveley, Hitchin, Herts SG4 7EQ
Tel: 01707 661005
(The foundation will supply information about animal healing, seminars, and clinics.)

Training in animal healing

UK

Self Realization Meditation Healing Centre

Laurel Lane, Queen Camel, Yeovil, Somerset BA22 7NU

Tel: 01935 850266

Fax: 01935 850234

E-mail: info@selfrealizationcentres.org

Internet: www.selfrealizationcentres.org

(Referral service and short courses in animal healing are open to anyone who wishes to learn about healing.)

Canada

Self Realization Meditation Healing Centre

RR9 736 Creekside Crescent, Gibsons Landing BC, VON 1V9

Tel: (604) 886 0898

(Animal healing courses and referral service.)

Australia

Self Realization Meditation Healing Centre

53 Regent Street, Paddington, 2021 NSW

Tel: 029 331 4656

Fax: 029 331 6701

New Zealand

Self Realization Meditation Healing Centre

100 Highsted Road, Bishopdale, Christchurch

Tel: 03 359 8507

Fax: 03 359 3430

2 Harbour View Road, PO Box 129, Leigh

Tel: 09 422 6363

Fax: 09 422 6368

CHAPTER THIRTEEN

Herbal medicine

AT-A-GLANCE GUIDE

What is it? The use of plants to restore health and heal disease.

What can it help? Most physical problems, some behavioural problems.

Can you do it yourself? Yes.

Average cost of treatment? Home-grown herbs and those growing wild are free! Bought herbs are relatively inexpensive. Veterinary treatment using herbs will be in line with standard veterinary fees, possibly more expensive depending on the length of consultation.

Is it safe? Yes, when used sensibly and in the correct dosage.

Herbal medicine uses plants to heal. It is an holistic treatment and takes account of the animal's whole being and the many factors that unite to cause illness, such as inadequate diet and stress. Herbal medicine is gentle and often slow-acting but supports and stimulates the body to self-heal, so the results are long-lasting and potentially curative.

Herbal medicine encompasses a range of well-known plants, some of which we eat regularly, like parsley and mint.

Using plants to heal

Herbal medicine is one of the oldest forms of healing and, despite domestication, animals instinctively know which herbs and plants will help them when they are ill. How often have you watched your dog or cat eating grass and then being sick? If they are feeling ill they look for plants that will purge their system; at other times they may eat plants to get extra nutrients. Nature provides us with all we need; it is just a question of knowing what to take.

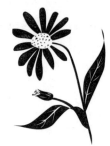

In the wild, animals usually eat the stomach contents of their prey first, because this is where the partially digested and highly nutritious plant material is. For the same reason, some dogs eat horse dung, especially when the grass is new because they know it is a rich and digestible source of nutrients. I often watch my own dog pottering around in the garden picking out different plants and grasses – and he always eats horse dung in the spring!

Many vets and pet owners are rediscovering the power of herbs, and as a result there are many different herbal remedies available – from fresh or dried herbs to tablets, ointments and tinctures.

How does it work?

Like other forms of natural medicine, herbs work in harmony with an animal's body and encourage it to self-heal and overcome illness. Because it is such an ancient form of medicine, the therapeutic plants are well-documented and most herbal remedies are used in low doses and side effects are rare.

Herbs contain a range of active constituents which help the body fight unwanted ailments. For example they can sedate overactive organs, relax tense muscles and nerves, stimulate circulation, strengthen tissues, revitalise the body, boost the immune system and reduce inflammation. Essentially, herbs support the body systems in fighting disease rather than just relieving the symptoms.

'Mammalian bodies are designed to live a healthy life – this is their natural state, this is their birthright – and the body has a tendency to make efforts to return to being healthy. So when you are looking at things holistically you are attempting to help the body to return to being healthy. You are also trying to remove the influences – medicinal, nutritional, or environmental – which are harmful and which lead to ill health.'

John Rohrbach, MVetMed, MRCVS

Using herbs with animals

In most cases the same herbs that are used for treating humans can also be used safely for dogs and cats, with a few exceptions. Cats are highly sensitive to some herbs and are affected differently from dogs. The herbs not to give cats are marigold, marijuana, cocoa, or white-willow bark. However, when in doubt check with your vet or a herbalist and stick to the commonly used herbs until you get more experienced.

Plants contain natural healing powers, and because of their long history we know which plants we can use safely and what effect they will have. For example, scullcap and valerian are commonly used for treating nervous problems in animals as they have a calming and sooth-ing effect, and psyllium husks are great for alleviating constipation. It is easy to forget that before modern medicine, herbal medicine was an every day way to cure ills.

Because of the popularity of fast-acting modern drugs, herbal medi-cine has taken a back seat but, as more and more people are concerned with the adverse side effects of many drugs and are wanting more natural treatments for themselves and their pets, herbal medicine is enjoying a great revival.

Can herbs be harmful?

Not everything that is natural is necessarily safe, and some herbs are toxic in large doses. Just because the side effects are minimal and instances of adverse reactions are rare, it does not mean that herbal medicines are completely safe to take. Herbs are powerful medicines and need to be treated with respect. Anything taken in excess or taken inappropriately may be detrimental.

Something you have to be careful of in herbal medicine is getting a diagnosis and then treating your animal yourself without veterinary supervision. Talk to your vet and say you want to try something other than drugs and most vets will be happy to refer you as long as they can keep their eye on the situation. You have to play safe with difficult conditions but anything that is not life-threatening you can treat your-self with herbs.

The answer is not to give anything if you do not know what it is or what it is expected to do.

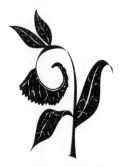

The healing properties of herbs

Herbal medicine covers a vast range of healing possibilities, from the mild-acting plant medi-cines like chamomile and peppermint to the very potent ones like pokeroot and wormwood. Herbs have different properties, ranging from nutritive to medicinal.

Herbs are easy to get hold of and come in many forms – fresh herbs, dried, tinctures, tablets, ointments, compresses, poultices, infu-sions, decoctions, oils, and capsules – and there are several herbal reme-dies specifically made for dogs and cats (see suppliers at end of chapter).

What can herbal medicine help?

It can help most physical illnesses and disorders, such as chronic, long-term problems like arthritis and rheumatism, and some of the more acute problems like kennel cough and other bacterial infections. Herbal remedies can also help with behavioural problems, such as anxiety and nervousness. Below is a guide to some of the conditions herbal medicine is effective in treating:

- Rheumatism, arthritis.
- Skin problems, such as eczema.
- Digestive problems, such as diarrhoea, constipation, colic, wind.
- Infections.
- Worms, parasites, fleas.
- Kidney conditions.
- Respiratory problems.
- Heart problems.
- Nervous conditions.

Herbal medicines can also be used for a wide range of minor problems that are easy to treat at home, including stomach upset, vomiting, constipation, diarrhoea, digestive problems, sore muscles, skin rashes, burns and allergies.

Properly used, herbs can have a gentle action and help the body to heal itself.

For specific ailments and first-aid use, see Chapters 16 and 17.

Consulting a herbal vet

If you wish to use herbal treatment for your pet but the case is too complicated or serious to treat safely at home, then get a referral to a vet who uses herbal treatments in their practice. (See useful information at the end of the chapter.)

> 'It is very important that if people do not want orthodox treatment and they want herbal treatment, they should say so to their vet. I have some vets who ask me to treat their own animals and some of them have come to thinking in this way because again and again they are hearing from clients who are interested in using herbs and they think there might be something in this.'
>
> *John Rohrbach, MVetMed, MRCVS*

> Selecting the right herbs for the problem can have a profound healing effect without the danger of side effects associated with many modern drugs.

> 'There are a variety of reasons that people ask me for herbal treatment for their pets. Some regard it as a natural form of medicine to be used. Others want to avoid continued orthodox treatment – repeated courses of antibiotics, steroids yet again, or even trying to avoid an operation. Some people have a knowledge of what herbs can do and they want it because they know it is a very effective form of treatment.'
>
> *John Rohrbach, MVetMed, MRCVS*

The healing action of herbs

Herbs are often categorised according to the kind of problem they will help. The right herb can be chosen by knowing what effect it will have on the body and what effect you are wanting.

Below is a list of some of the actions herbs have that makes them beneficial for healing disease:

- Anthelminitic herbs destroy or expel intestinal worms, eg wormwood, garlic, black walnut.
- Anti-inflammatory herbs soothe and reduce inflammation, eg chamomile, wild yam.
- Anti-microbial herbs strengthens the body's resistance to infections and in general aid the body's natural immunity to disease, eg clove, eucalyptus.
- Anti-spasmodic herbs prevent and ease cramps or spasms in the body, eg cramp bark, chamomile.
- Astringent herbs can reduce irritation and inflammation and create a barrier against infection that is helpful to wounds and burns, eg witch hazel.
- Bitter herbs have a special role in preventative medicine and stimulate appetite, aid the liver in detoxification and stimulate gut-healing, eg wormwood, barberry.
- Carminative herbs stimulate the digestive system and soothe the gut wall. They reduce any inflammation, ease griping pains and help to get rid of gas in the digestive tract, eg ginger, peppermint.
- Demulcent herbs soothe and protect irritated or inflamed tissue especially in the bowel; they help prevent diarrhoea and reduce the muscle spasms that cause colic, eg slippery elm.
- Laxative herbs promote bowel movement, eg cascara, senna.
- Nervine herbs help to strengthen and tone the nervous system. Some act as stimulants and some as relaxants, eg scullcap and valerian.
- Stimulating herbs invigorate the physio-logical and metabolic activity of the body, eg mustard and cayenne.
- Vulnerary herbs are applied externally and help to heal wounds and cuts, eg aloe vera, comfrey.

Treating your pet at home

One of the best uses for herbs is as a preventative measure – *before* health problems appear. Because they strengthen and tone, herbs can be part of your pet's natural diet throughout their life and help to keep them healthy and strong.

There may be times when you need to use fast-acting medical drugs, but when there is no danger to the animal, herbs make powerful healing agents. In many of the chronic cases, such as arthritis, herbs can often replace drugs entirely, although reduction of medication should only be done under the supervision of a vet. Many people prefer using whole plant remedies to avoid any adverse side effects that may be found with modern drugs.

Herbal medicine is also helpful in day-to-day first-aid treatment for things like cuts, burns and bites. Any first-aid treatment should be short-lived. If there is no improvement fairly quickly, then take your pet to the vet.

Keep in mind that, although herbs are gentle and safe, they are medicines and should be treated with respect. Always stick to the tried and tested remedies, or consult a herbal vet for more complicated cases. When buying herbs make sure they are from a reputable source, since the quality of the herbs used will determine their therapeutic potential.

Cost and availability

Freshly picked herbs cost nothing and you can grow your own. Otherwise, herbs and herbal products are relatively cheap and come in many forms. They are readily available in health-food shops, pharmacies, herbalists or by mail order (see suppliers at end of chapter).

How to use herbs for healing

Herbs can be taken internally or used externally on wounds. They make great first-aid remedies – within half an hour they can be boiled up and ready to use as a poultice or compress. If you have ointments, tinctures, pills or capsules to hand they can be used immediately.

One of the easiest ways to use herbal treatment is to get the ready-prepared ones for dogs and cats which come in tablets, tinctures and lotions. They always have instructions for use which makes them a good starting point until you feel ready to branch out and prepare your own. Once you feel more confident about using herbs for healing it is fun to collect and prepare them yourself and you will get great joy and satis-faction finding out more about herbal medicine and harvesting nature's healing garden.

Preparing your own herbs

You can either grow your own in the garden or in pots on a window sill, or gather herbs growing wild like nettles and dandelions. Try not to pick herbs that are growing too near a road as these will be polluted. Freshly picked herbs should be used fairly soon after picking or frozen for later use. Dried herbs will last for about a year as long as they are completely dry before storing. The best way to store dried herbs is in a dark glass jar or in a brown paper bag and keep them in a cool dark place.

Freshly picked herbs These can be chopped up and put straight into your pet's food eg parsley, garlic, dandelion.

Dried herbs These can be sprinkled on food eg nettle, comfrey, echinacea. Or made into a tea. Dried herbs can also be ground into a powder using a coffee grinder.

Infusion or tea You can make a tea from plant leaves and small stems by soaking 1 teaspoon of dried herbs (or 2 teaspoons of fresh herbs) in a cup of boiling water and leaving it for 20–30 minutes. The strained liquid will keep in the fridge for a few days. This is a good way of using common garden herbs like nettles, parsley and dandelions. Always use distilled or filtered water. The correct dosage of herb tea can be mixed into your pet's food or given in a dropper bottle straight into their mouth. Tilt their head back a little so that the liquid runs down their throat.

Decoction This is a tea made from roots, bark, stems, or seeds. Put 1 rounded teaspoon (or 3 fresh herbs) of the crushed or chopped herb into water and simmer gently for about 30 minutes. Leave it to cool, strain and use as an infusion. This will last a few days in the fridge. Always use distilled or filtered water and a non-aluminium pan. This can be given in the same way as for a herb tea.

Capsules These contain powdered herbs and can be given with or without food. If your pet won't take capsules, you can open them up and tip the contents into their food.

Tablets Powdered herbs. These can be taken with or without food and crushed to make them easier to take.

Tinctures Herbs that have been preserved in alcohol or some other pre-serving agent, such as vegetable glycerine, are called tinctures. They come in dropper bottles and can be easily placed into an animal's mouth or added to their food. Tinctures are easy to use and they last for several years without losing their potency. (It is best not to use tinctures preserved in alcohol when treating pets with any kind of liver disease.)

External use
Ointments Herbal ointments, such as calendula and comfrey, are good for cuts and wounds.

Poultice A poultice of fresh herbs can be useful in a first-aid situation. To make a poultice, mash fresh plants with a little boiling water to make a paste. This can be placed on the affected area when still hot, but not boiling, and covered with a piece of gauze.

Compress These can be used hot or cold. A hot compress helps to bring heat to the area in order to kill germs, stimulate drainage and relax muscles. Soak a clean cloth in a herbal tea and apply hot (not boiling) to the infected area. Cover it with a dry towel to keep the heat in. After five minutes refresh the compress and reapply. You can do this for 15 minutes if your pet will let you, twice a day for up to two weeks. Hot and cold compresses can be alternated to stimulate blood supply to the area.

Soaking Make a warm infusion and immerse the animal's leg, tail or foot in the liquid for at least five minutes before drying. This can be done twice a day for up to two weeks.

Powders Golden seal powder for infections and cuts; witch hazel to stop bleeding of minor wounds.

Length of treatment
It really depends on what is being treated. For example an acute, short-term condition like diarrhoea can respond very quickly; whereas a longer-term chronic condition like arthritis can take much longer to respond. In general, only allow a day for an acute illness and two to three weeks for chronic problems before any great improvement can be seen. When in doubt consult your vet or a medical herbalist.

Dosage
It is important to give the correct dosage since herbal medicine works best used correctly. More does not mean better results and could be dangerous.

For acute conditions
Cats and small dogs 1/4 teaspoon of an infusion or decoction 3 times a day or 2 drops of tincture. Tiny pinch of dried herbs or 1/2 teaspoon of fresh herbs.

Medium dogs 1/2 teaspoon of an infusion or decoction 3 times a day or 5 drops of tincture. A pinch of dried herbs or 3/4 teaspoon of fresh herbs.

Large dogs 1 to 2 teaspoons of infusion or decoction 3 times a day or 9 drops of tincture. 1/2 teaspoon of dried herbs or 1 teaspoon of fresh herbs.

This can be given until the symptoms disappear or for a maximum of a week. If there is still no improvement consult your vet. The capsules and tablets made specifically for dogs and cats have instructions for use on the container. When using your own herbs, fresh or dried, they can be mixed into your pet's food.

For chronic conditions
Use the same dosage as above but continue for 8 to 12 weeks.

Response to treatment
The action of herbal treatment can be so gentle that you may think nothing is happening, but be patient and watch your pet carefully so that you notice any changes as these will help you to decide what effect treatment is having and whether to continue it, stop it or try something else.

One of the first signs that the treatment is working is the animal seems 'more like itself', with better energy and better mood. Physical improvements can often be slower to occur so be aware of possible psychological changes. Sometimes there may be a healing reaction, such as a discharge, which is another sign that healing is taking place. A healing reaction is usually short-lived but if you are in any doubt whether your animal is getting worse, call the vet. It can take time for poisons to be eliminated from an animal's system and for strength and vitality to return.

Herbal medicine chest for cats and dogs

Aloe vera Healing agent. Taken internally (liquid) for a wide range of digestive complaints, as a general tonic and for its cleansing properties. Used externally (gel or spray) on burns, cuts, wounds, insect bites and skin irritations. Aloe vera soothes inflamed skin, protects against infection and speeds the healing process. If you have an aloe

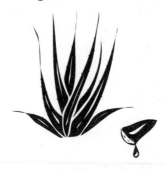

vera plant, break off part of the leaf and apply the aloe gel directly to the affected part. Aloe vera has powerful anti-inflammatory and antiseptic properties. It also helps to regenerate tissue at the cellular level.

Astragalus Chinese herb. One of the most effective herbs for supporting the immune system. Available fresh, dried, tablets and tincture.

Cat's claw Antioxidant, detoxifying, anti-microbial, anti-inflammatory and boosts the immune system. It increases stamina and energy in animals suffering physical and mental exhaustion and balances emotions in cases of extreme stress. Taken internally for a wide range of illnesses including cancer, bowel problems and skin complaints. Cat's claw can be used in capsule form or taken as a tea.

Comfrey Healing agent. Helps to heal bones. It can be taken internally or used as a cream. Good for bruises, cuts and wounds.

Echinacea Fights infections; boosts the immune system, reduces allergic reactions. It can be used externally as a tincture (diluted in water) to promote the healing of cuts and various skin irritations. Available as capsules, dried herbs, tablets and tincture.

Eye bright Eye problems. Can be take internally or used externally as soothing eye wash to alleviate inflammation.

Garlic Antiseptic, anti-fungal, anti-viral, anti-bacterial properties. Effective in treating parasites and infections. Helps to boost the immune system. Best used fresh and raw, or in capsule form if your pet does not like the taste of fresh garlic.

Ginger Soothing to the digestive system. Good for indigestion and wind. Also a warming herb and helps circulation problems and arthritis. Helpful for relieving travel sickness. Commonly used fresh or as capsules.

Milk thistle Restores liver function and is supportive and reparative. It reduces the toxic effects of conventional drugs and helps the liver to detoxify. Good for animals that have been receiving a lot of veterinary treatment, such as drugs, chemotherapy, vaccinations, worming tablets etc. It cleanses and repairs the liver and is a helpful addition to a pet's diet where detoxification is needed. Available as capsules, tablets and tincture.

Psyllium husks For cleansing the bowel and alleviating constipation. Used as capsules or loose.

Slippery elm Soothing. Good for digestive problems and stomach pains. Tablets or powder.

Witch hazel Reduces inflammation and irritation; protects against infection. Used externally on wounds and burns. It can also be used powdered or as a cream.

Herbs in the diet

Small quantities of commonly used culinary herbs like thyme, marjoram, sage, rosemary, parsley, dandelion, nettle and watercress are useful additions to the diet. They have health-giving properties in themselves and are good sources of minerals, vitamins and trace elements. Nettles, for example, are rich in vitamin C and iron, parsley is high in vitamin C, and kelp contains a wide range of essential elements. You can mix a few herbs together in a container and sprinkle a small pinch of the mixed herbs on your pet's food a few times a week. Cats and dogs will naturally go out and chew on herbs – it is all part of a good, healthy, balanced diet.

Herbal medicine has a place in modern veterinary practice and is regaining its traditional place in many surgeries for the treatment of common and chronic complaints.

Can herbs be given at the same time as other treatments?

In general they can be given along with standard veterinary treatment and some of the complementary treatments like acupuncture and chiropractic. However, some people would say not to give strong-smelling herbs like garlic and peppermint at the same time as homoeopathic remedies or flower remedies since the herbs can affect these and cause them to lose their potency. It is usually a good idea to give one type of natural treatment a chance to work before adding another one.

Case history: a cat with fleas and an allergy to flea bites

'Ferdinand is a large tabby and white cat. He was infested with fleas. In addition he had the typical scabby skin lesions that result from an allergy to flea bites. His owner had been taking him to the local vet for treatment, and she had been supplied with two toxic chemical sprays: one to use on Ferdie and the other to be sprayed around the house. In addition the vet had been treating him with corticosteriods to reduce the symptoms of allergy. Ferdie's owners did not think this was the best or, indeed, the safest course of action, either for Ferdie or for the human inhabitants of the house.

'She asked for a referral to this practice for herbal treatment. With a problem like this it was necessary to do more than simply use a herbal medicine: a more holistic approach was necessary. So other treatments and measures were advised in addition to the herbal treatment.

'Herbal treatment was sent in the form of a liquid medication to be given by mouth. This consisted of extracts in diluted glycerin of: burdock root, yellow dock root, chebulic myrobalan fruit, emblic myrobalan fruit, liquorice root, fenugreek seed and southern-wood leaf.

'The treatment with corticosteroids had only been intermittent and the cat had not had any for several weeks, so it was necessary to arrange for a gradual reduction in the dosage of this medication. (If treatment with corticosteroids has been given at sufficient dosage over a period of time the patient's adrenal glands atrophy, with the result that their ability to produce the natural hormones is reduced. Sudden cessation of treatment in this situation could put the patient at risk of a life-threatening illness, particularly if any other condition or accident occurred in the ensuing weeks.)

'Dietary supplements of capsules containing natural vitamin E and capsules of evening primrose oil and fish oils were supplied. His diet was improved by ceasing dry food and a poor-quality tinned food; he was instead fed tinned food made from a reputable manufacturer. Later, some cooked mashed vegetables were added to this.

'Advice was given about how to reduce the reinfestation from hatching fleas in the house by vacuum cleaning. In view of the tender and irritated state of his skin, no medication was used against fleas; however, he was groomed gently once daily and attempts were to be made to catch and kill any fleas that could be found.

'A few weeks later a very dilute suspension of tea tree oil was supplied. This was sprinkled over the coat before grooming. Soon there was a reduction in the intensity and amount of skin licking and scratching that Ferdie was doing; the scabs disappeared and his fur started to grow.

'In subsequent years his owner has phoned when the symptoms reappear. The same treatment, but without the tea tree oil, has been sent and within two weeks he has improved.'

©1997 John A. Rohrbach, MVetMed, MRCVS

Useful information

Where to find a herbal vet
UK
The British Association of Homoeopathic Veterinary Surgeons
Chinham House, Stanford-in-the-Vale, Faringdon, Oxon SN7 8NQ
Tel: 01367 718115
Internet: www.bahvs.com
(Send a sae for list of vets using herbal remedies.)

John A. Rohrbach MVetMed, MRCVS
Ard-Laggan, Perth Road, Crieff, Perthshire PH7 3EQ
Tel: 01764 653320

US
American Holistic Veterinary Medicine Association
2214 Old Emmorton Road, Bel Air, Maryland 21015
Tel: (410) 569 0795
Fax: (410) 515 7774
(Call or write, sending a sae, for a list of vets who are members in your area.)

Australia
Holistic Animal Therapy Association of Australia
PO Box 202, Ormond, Victoria 3204
Tel/Fax: (03) 9578 3710

Suppliers of herbs and herbal products for dogs and cats
UK
Hilton Herbs Ltd
Downclose Farm, North Perrott, Crewkerne, Somerset TA18 7SH
Tel: 01460 78300
Fax: 01460 78302
(Suppliers of a wide range of herbs and herbal products such as garlic powder and granules, seaweed, slippery elm, echinacea as well as ready-prepared mixes such as canine coat and skin, canine endurance, canine temperament and comfrey compress. They also supply a range of other products, such as comfrey oil, flower remedies, magnetic rugs, homoeopathic remedies etc.)

Dorwest Herbs
Shipton George, Bridport, Dorset DT6 4LP
Tel: 01308 897272
Fax: 01308 897929
E-mail: dorwest@cix.compulink.co.uk
(Suppliers of ready-made herbal tablets for dogs and cats.)

Hambleden Herbs
Court Farm, Milverton, Somerset TA4 1NF
Tel: 01823 401104
Fax: 01823 401001
Email: info@hambledenherbs.co.uk
Internet: www.hambledenherbs.co.uk
(Suppliers of organic herbs.)

Acorn Supplements Ltd,
(See Chapter 5 for details.)

Faithful Friends
(See Chapter 5 for details.)

US
Crystal Star Herbal Nutrition
4069 Wedge Way Court, Earth City, MO 63045
Tel: (800) 736 6015
(Suppliers of herbal combination remedies for people and pets. They claim to have a ready-made herb for just about every ailment.)

Healing Herbs for Pets
Tel: (888) 775 7387
(Offers a complete line of Chinese herbs for pets.)

Ambrican Enterprises, Ltd.
PO Box 1436, Jacksonville, OR 97530
Tel: (541) 899-2080
Fax: (541) 899-3414
Email: ambrican@cdsnet.net
(Natural supplements, herbs, and importers of Juliette de Bairacli Levy's Natural Rearing herbal products for dogs and cats.)

CHAPTER FOURTEEN

Homoeopathy

AT-A-GLANCE GUIDE

What is it? Minute doses of natural substances usually given in tablet form. Works on the principle of 'like cures like'.

What can it help? Most physical diseases, mental and emotional problems, injuries and bruising.

Can you do it yourself? Yes.

Average cost of the remedies? The remedies cost just a few pounds, and are widely available.

Average cost of treatment by a homoeopathic vet? In line with standard veterinary fees. However, the extra time involved can mean it is more expensive, in line with referral fees.

Homoeopathy is one of the most popular complementary treatments for animals and many vets use it in their practice. It lends itself particularly well to home use since the remedies are simple to use, easy to get hold of and inexpensive.

Homoeopathy is an holistic treatment and treats each animal as an individual. It is just as effective on cats and dogs as it is with people and they generally respond well, disproving any claims of a placebo effect. It is a gentle treatment for animals and allows them to heal from the inside out.

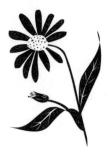

How it began

Although the 'similia principle' (like cures like) dates back hundreds of years BC it was only redis-covered about 200 years ago by a German doctor, Samuel Hahnemann, who went on to build up a repertoire of diseases and remedies. While conventional medicine treats illness with an antidote, homoeopathy treats illness with a similar substance, only potentised. Hahnemann developed the potentising of natural substances to avoid harmful side effects. He also discovered that homoeopathy treats the whole being and works just as well with emotional and mental problems as it does with physical disease.

How does it work?

Homoeopathy is an energy medicine and, just like the flower essences, acupuncture and healing, it has a positive effect on the animal's vital force. Homoeopathy sees symptoms of disease as a disturbance of the vital force and therefore by positively stimulating it, the animal's own powers of self-healing are set in motion. In short, it encourages the body to behave in a more healthy way.

Homoeopathy works on the principle of 'like cures like' in the sense that a substance that can cause symptoms of illness can also be used in a potentised form to treat those symptoms. For example, a fever similar to belladonna poisoning could be cured by potentised belladonna.

Like the flower essences, homoeopathic remedies do not contain any material or physical amount of the original substance. The substance is diluted over and over again until only its energy or vibration is left. The more diluted the substance is, the more far-reaching is its healing potential.

Homoeopathy does not treat the disease, it treats the animal with the disease.

Using homoeopathy with animals

One of the biggest moving forces behind bringing homoeopathy into modern veterinary use was the British vet, the late George MacLeod, who wrote numerous books on treating animals with homoeopathy, from goats and horses to cats and dogs. It has since become one of the most widely used natural medicines for treating animals. Because is it harmless and simple to use it has also become one of the most popular remedies to use at home.

Making a diagnosis

The key to successful treatment lies in getting the right match for the animal's symptoms with the properties of the remedy. When building a 'picture' of the disease homoeopathy takes account of:

- the actual signs or symptoms, which might be diarrhoea, sickness and lethargy,
- the length of time they have been ill,
- the general constitutional type of the animal (for example, a labrador is prone to being slow and fat whereas a setter is bouncy and lively),
- the individual characteristics of the animal,
- the modalities – better or worse when hot or cold, better or worse with movement,
- odd characteristics, such as a fever but no thirst.

Once you have a 'disease picture' you can choose the right homoeo-pathic remedy. When treating less complicated cases this is fairly easy to do and many of the remedies suit particular symptoms, such as arnica for bruising or aconite for shock. In cases like this the diagnosis is simple, and very often you will be able to treat your cat or dog effectively your-self and recovery can be rapid. Sometimes though, the situation may be too complicated to manage by yourself, in which case it is best to seek the advice of an experienced homoeopathic vet. See Where to find a homoeopathic vet at the end of the chapter.

'It is not always easy to see the true picture. In general, the more drug treatment an animal has had the more confused the picture of disease is. Homoeopathy often works stage by stage, like peeling the layers off an onion, where you treat the symptoms you see to start with and then, as the symptoms change, the animal is still ill, but you treat the new picture. You're peeling back layers of an onion until you get to the essential problem and it can take time to get to the heart of it.'

June Third-Carter, VetMFHom

Consulting a homoeopathic vet

There are many vets who practise homoeopathy and details of how to find one are given at the end of the chapter.

Appointments can take up to half an hour, during which the homoeopath will want to amass as much information as possible about the animal to build up a picture of the disease.

Healing reactions

Homoeopathic remedies stimulate and support the body's own healing mechanism and sometimes this leads to an 'aggravation' or flare-up of symptoms. If a remedy is spot-on and fits the picture accurately, the animal can get a brief increase in the severity of the symptoms. An itchy rash will become a horrendously itchy rash, and an animal suffering from a digestive problem may get a bout of diarrhoea. In homoeopathy this is seen as a good sign, because it shows the remedy is working and that the animal's natural forces of recovery are in action. The aggravations show that the remedy is having a spring-cleaning effect. Healing reactions like these are usually quick to pass and should not be treated, or suppressed, as they are an important part of the healing process.

'I believe homoeopathy is a purer form of medicine than allopathy but both have their uses.'

June Third-Carter, VetMFHom

The remedies

The remedies come from plant, animal or mineral sources, such as poppies, toad poison and oyster shells. They are made by qualified pharmacists and are produced by diluting the original substance in water or alcohol often thousands of times and shaking it vigorously to release its curative energy. This process makes even poisonous substances perfectly safe to use.

The remedies are made in different potencies or dilutions. The potencies are always indicated on the container and come in dilutions of tens, hundreds or thousands. A ten-times dilution is marked with an x, a hundred-times dilution is marked with a c, and a thousand-times dilution is marked with an m. Mostly with animals you will be using lower potencies of 6c or 30c and these are the ones you will find in pharmacists and health-food stores.

High or low potencies are not stronger or weaker in the normal sense, but more like different radio frequencies – a low potency carries a wide range and will help even if it is not spot on. A high potency carries a much narrower range so that it must be spot on to have an effect – and the effect can last for months or years.

Remedies are usually sold in tablet form, tiny sugar-milk pellets which can be easily crushed and placed on an animal's tongue. Other forms of homoeopathic medicine include ointments, tinctures, powders, and creams.

Are they safe?

For first-aid use in the low potencies the remedies are perfectly safe and you can not overdose with them in the same way as you can with medical drugs. Quantity makes no difference to the overall effect. Whether you take 100 tablets or one tablet the effect will be the same. If it is the right remedy the effect will be positive; if it is the wrong remedy nothing will happen. Giving more than the required dose is just a waste, since it won't have an enhanced effect.

With very deep-seated or long-term ailments continued use of the wrong remedy, where no positive effects are being observed, can muddy the picture or stall the healing process. In cases like this, it's best to consult a homoeopathic vet.

What can it help?

Because homoeopathy is an holistic treatment and treats the whole being, it can have a therapeutic effect on almost any problem as long as the right remedy is used. You could say that homoeopathy works well for almost any condition, but not for every animal. When an animal does not respond to a remedy there can be a number of reasons why, including the wrong remedy having been given or if the picture is muddled by a history of drug treatment or a strong family history of a problem.

Minor, short-term, acute problems respond well. These include diarrhoea, constipation, bee stings, bruising, allergies and vomiting.

Chronic, long-term conditions that respond well include skin problems, arthritis, diabetes, emotional disorders, epilepsy.

In homoeopathy – treat the animals and it will fight the disease itself.

For specific ailments and first-aid use, see Chapters 16 and 17.

Case histories

'A good indication of how quickly a remedy can work is the case of a collapsed dog that I went out to see on a house call. The dog was cold and its pulse was weak. I gave it aconite and by the time I had driven back to the surgery it was up on its feet. So that is a good illustration of giving aconite for shock.'

'I had a dog with a skin problem that was really stumping me until I examined his mother. She always had skin trouble and I was able to see a clearer 'picture' with her and worked out the remedy that way. I just couldn't get it from seeing him but I got it from seeing the mother's constitution. Long-term things like that coming through the generations often can't be cured but they can be eased.'

'Ginger was a 14-year-old cat with liver failure who came to see me. He was emaciated, jaundiced, off his food and had a very swollen liver. With a mixture of phosphorus and ptelea he regained his appetite within 48 hours and steadily recovered over a month and had no further problems. Before this he was on antibiotics and steroids and he had been deteriorating rapidly.'

June Third-Carter, VetMFHom

Advantages of treating homoeopathically

As with other forms of natural medicine, by treating your pet with homoeopathy you have the chance of getting a complete cure because it is getting to the root cause of the problem and leaving the animal stronger afterwards. A long course of antibiotics or steroids, by contrast, will leave the animal weakened. Although modern drugs relieve pain and stop infections, they also have side effects. In the end they leave the animal in a weaker position and so there is more likely to be trouble in the future, but you may get the animal through a crisis.

'Very often if you're suppressing or apparently curing something superficial you are actually going to get something deeper next time. Say treating anal glands with antibiotics then the animal can develop a chronic enteritis afterwards. One disease follows on from another once you start using drugs.'

June Third-Carter, VetMFHom

Home use

There are thousands of different homoeopathic remedies, but don't panic – you won't have to become familiar with them all! Certain remedies work for a variety of common complaints and make up a good, all-round medicine chest to use at home. Always seek veterinary help in serious cases or if your animal is suffering a lot of pain.

All homoeopathic remedies have Latin names but are commonly known by their abbreviated versions. For example calcarea carbonica is known as calc. carb. and rhus toxicodendron is known as rhus tox.

There are several very good books on homoeopathy for animals which will give you further insights into using this form of natural medicine.

Buying the remedies

Each remedy is clearly labelled and will have its abbreviated Latin name marked on the container, along with its strength or potency. For example, rhus tox. 6c, calc. carb. 30c. (See the end of the chapter for suppliers.)

They come in tiny sugar-milk tablets which are easy for animals to take and some manufacturers make soft tablets specially for animals.

The remedies come in a range of different potencies, but when treating animals 6c strength is the best one to use. A homoeopathic vet may well use much stronger remedies, but unless you are experienced it is best to stick to 6c or 30c with your own pet.

Dosage

The amount given for cats and dogs is the same as for people since size is not an important factor. The frequency of the dose is very important and depends on whether the disease is chronic or acute.

In urgent, acute cases

Give 1 tablet every 15 to 20 minutes for the first 3 hours, then 1 tablet every hour for the rest of the day. After that give 1 tablet 3 times a day for a few more days or until the symptoms have disappeared.

If it is something that is very severe, give the remedy and, if you are not getting an improvement in an hour or two, go to the vet. In less severe cases, if there is no change at all within 24 hours then you could try a different remedy. It is important to watch your pet's reaction after they take the remedy, since any change is a sign that healing is taking place and often they will become very relaxed and go to sleep.

Do not keep trying different remedies, if your pet does not respond to one or two in the first few days then seek professional help. Common sense must be applied when dealing with acute cases.

In chronic cases

Give 1 tablet 3 times a day for a week, then 1 tablet twice a day for another few weeks. If the problem is very long-term then 1 tablet a week for several weeks will be enough. Often results can come long after the remedy has been given and, as a rule of thumb, the longer a condition has been going on the longer it will take to heal. It is a case of being patient and watching carefully for any changes on any level.

If your animal does get an aggravation, stop the remedy for about 24 hours and start it again once it has calmed down. If it does not calm down either wait a bit longer (if the animal is not suffering in any way) or use strong peppermint or coffee as an antidote. Remember an aggravation is a good sign and shows that you have the right remedy. A severe aggravation is unlikely with low potencies, but never risk an aggravation with a very weak or old animal, because it (and you) may not be able to cope.

Giving the remedies

Due to their fragile nature there are some important guidelines to follow when using homoeopathic remedies:

- Do not touch the remedies. Put them straight into the animal's mouth on the container lid or from a plastic spoon.
- If your pet resists taking the remedy (cats often do) you can crush it up in a small amount of milk or some butter or anything else your pet relishes, including ice cream!
- Give the remedies away from meals, leaving about half an hour before or after a meal time.
- If you are using more than one type of remedy at a time, separate them by at least five minutes.

Storing the remedies

By the very nature of homoeopathic remedies being an energetic form of medicine, this also makes them fragile and easily damaged. However, if you keep to the following guidelines they should last for quite a few years:

- Store the remedies away from strong smells, such as peppermint, camphor, perfume.
- Store in a dark cupboard, keep away from strong light.
- Store at room temperature.
- Keep the lid on when not in use.

Is homoeopathy compatible with other treatments?

Because homoeopathy is an holistic way by treating the animal as a whole, it should be given a chance to work on its own before adding other forms of medicine. It complements well some of the more physical treatments and remedies such as conventional veterinary care, chiropractic, herbs and nutrition, but try not to mix it with other energy medicines like acupuncture or healing, as they can interfere with each other.

Homoeopathic alternatives to vaccinations

See Chapter 6.

Homoeopathic medicine chest for cats and dogs

The following remedies make up a basic medicine chest for healing simple day-to-day complaints. It is a good idea to buy these in advance so that you have them to hand when you need them.

Aconite For shock, fear and the start of any condition.
Keynote – sudden.

Arnica The first remedy to reach for in cases of bruising, shock, accident, or injury and for stings, sprains and strained muscles. It also helps with post-operative bruising. You can also use arnica ointment, but not on broken skin.
Keynote – 'ouch!'

Belladonna For fevers. If the animal is very hot with dilated pupils, use this fever remedy rather than aconite. It is the main remedy for fevers with redness, heat and dilated pupils. For heatstroke and great thirst.
Keynote – hot.

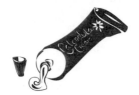

Calendula cream For minor cuts and grazes, scratches and wounds. Can be used where the skin has broken. Calendula cream is often combined with hypericum for pain relief.

Gelsemium Nervousness is the main use, along with anticipatory fear.
Keynote – trembling.

Hepar. sulph. For abscesses, cat bites, coughs, blocked anal glands, or when the glands are up in the neck. Use hepar sulph if you think puss is starting to form, or the area is looking swollen, red or painful. If there is a sudden discharge. For infected wounds which are producing pus. For infected ears where there is a discharge.
Keynote – very sore, smelly.

Hypericum Known as the 'homoeopathic painkiller'. Used for injuries where the nerves are affected, post-operative pain, spinal injuries, wounds with shooting pains, puncture wounds, injuries to toes and tails. Can also use hypericum ointment.
Keynote – pain.

Mercury Some diarrhoeas, infections in the mouth, bleeding discharge from the gums, flat teeth that are going to need some dentistry as well

to calm the gums down, pus-filled eyes. Also for some discharges, if it is very red and sore.
Keynote – ulcers, smelly.

Nux vomica For digestive upsets, wind, travel sickness, indigestion, some diarrhoeas, vomiting and irritability.
Keynote – irritable, chilly.

Rhus tox For spotty rashes, lameness that is worse just after rest, but improves after moving, sprains and strains. For rheumatism, arthritis and general joint pains that are better for movement. Also for acute skin problems.
Keynote – spotty, better for movement.

Sulphur Some diarrhoeas, skin problems, or if you feel an animal is just a bit run down, sulphur is a useful course of treatment.
Keynote – worse for heat.

As you get more experienced you can start adding more remedies to your core stock.

When using homoeopathy at home remember to be patient and give the chosen remedy a chance to work before moving onto another one. A lot depends on the condition you are treating, but if you use too many remedies at a time the picture can get muddled and it's hard to know what is working and what isn't. In homoeopathy, *more is not better*; one remedy given at the correct intervals with a large portion of patience is the best way!

'I think homoeopathy for animals is becoming more accepted – or more demanded – now. People are curious. A lot of people expect it to do miracles; it doesn't always, but it can be really satisfying to work with.'

June Third-Carter, VetFMHom

Useful information

Where to find a homoeopathic vet
UK
The British Association of Homoeopathic Veterinary Surgeons
Chinham House, Stanford-in-the-Vale, Faringdon, Oxon SN7 8NQ
Tel: 01367 718115
Internet: www.bahvs.com
(Send a sae for list of registered homoeopathic vets.)

US
National Centre for Homoeopathy
801 N. Fairfax #306, Alexandria, VA 22314
Tel: (703) 548 7790
Email: info@homeopathic.org

Australia
Holistic Animal Therapy Association of Australia
PO Box 202, Ormond, Victoria 3204
Tel/Fax: (03) 9578 3710

Where to buy homoeopathic remedies
Pharmacists and health-food stores

Mail order
UK
Ainsworths Homoeopathic Pharmacy
36 New Cavendish Street, London W1M 7LH
Tel: 0201 935 5330
Fax: 0201 486 4313
E-mail: Ainshom@msn.com
Internet: www.Ainsworths.com

Weleda UK Ltd
Heanor Road, Ilkeston, Derbyshire DE7 8DR
Tel: 01159 448200
Fax: 01159 448210
Internet: www.eweleda.co.uk

US

Botanical Laboratories, Inc.
1441 West Smith Road, Ferndale, WA 98248
Tel: (800) 232 4005
(Suppliers of homoeopathic remedies for people and pets.)

Dr Goodpet
PO Box 4547, Inglewood, CA 90309
Tel: (800) 222 9932
(Suppliers of homoeopathic remedies for animals.)

T-touch massage

T-touch is a way of healing and training animals using touch and body work. It was first developed in Canada by Linda Tellington-Jones, an animal behaviourist, and has since become popular as a treatment for pets. One of the major benefits of T-touch is that anyone can learn to do it – which makes it a great healing method for treating pets at home.

What is it?
T-touch is a way of working non-habitually with an animal's body to change habitual patterns of behaviour. This makes it a very effective

therapy for treating behavioural problems. It is based on Feldenkrais work on humans, which was developed by a man called Dr Moshe. He discovered that by using his body non-habitually – for example, getting another person to move his body in a non-habitual way, such as circling the leg in a way that he could not do on his own – he was able to create new neural pathways. These new pathways could bypass damaged neural pathways. Dr Moshe found that, by using this method of treatment, he recovered from an old injury that was inhibiting his walking.

Linda Tellington-Jones trained with Dr Moshe and realised the great potential the treatment had for healing animals. She first started using it for horses and then for all animals, dogs and cats, tigers, coyotes, leopards, birds, even whales!

T-touch is a way of working with and training an animal without using fear or force. It is a way of increasing intelligence because it creates new neural pathways. It can change an animal's posture and once you change the posture, you change the behaviour. T-touch combines touch, body-work movements and exercises to alter the whole pattern of behaviour of the animal.

How does it work?

It is thought that by opening up new nerve pathways using non-habitual massage movements, the brain can be activated into changing old habits and negative patterns of behaviour. T-touch body work is a way of stimulating cellular intelligence and thereby influencing the whole being of the animal – mind, body and spirit. It can bring about behavioural and personality changes and stimulate the healing of wounds, and injuries.

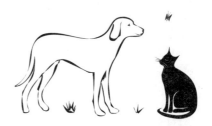

T-touch eases physical tension in the body and opens the neural pathways so that trapped emotions can also be released. Often an animal may become ill as a result of long-held emotions and unpleasant memories.

One of the most important aspects of using T-touch to heal is that it increases the communication between people and their pets. Touch is a powerful therapeutic tool and, used with T-touch, both humans and animals can reach greater levels of understanding each other. This non-verbal way of communicating with animals through mindful touch is at the heart of what T-touch is all about. It has been described as allowing you to 'open your heart and speak with your hands'.

Using T-touch with animals

T-touch is a wonderful treatment for animals because it is gentle and effective and strengthens the human-animal bond. It is also harmless and easy to learn.

T-touch involves using repeated, random massage movements over an animal's body. It is different from massage in its intent, which is to wake up the nervous system and make connections between the brain and the body. In a series of small circular movements the animal's skin is gently pushed in one and a quarter circles. The circles are made randomly all over the animal's body. This random way of working makes the animal's system wake up and pay attention, inviting movement opportunities the body had not previously thought of or experienced. It is thought that the brain pays attention to something that it is not familiar with, and this allows change to take place on all levels.

T-touch also involves ground-work exercises, depending on the nature of the problem. This may be leading an animal through a specific exercise course which helps them to focus, rebalance and listen to what is being asked of them.

What can be treated?

- All sorts of behavioural problems, such as aggression and excessive barking.
- Helpful in training situations and getting rid of bad habits.
- Minor injuries and wounds.
- Many physical problems, especially musculo-skeletal problems and inhibited mobility.
- Pain relief.
- Emotional problems, such as fear, nervousness, anxiety.

For specific ailments, see Chapter 17.

Case histories

'I have worked with aggressive dogs that have become docile, nervous dogs that have become courageous, horses that buck and bite and then stop doing it. T-touch can relieve pain and take away the fear that is trapped within an animal's body and therefore their behaviour completely changes.'

Sarah Fisher, T-touch practitioner

'I treated a dog, an eleven-year-old standard poodle, that had a rear leg ligament injury. The vet said that he thought the dog would have to be put down eventually because the good leg was going to give way. The dog was compensating by taking his weight off the bad leg and standing on the good leg. He could only lie on one side and he would growl in his sleep. He wasn't able to lift his leg to urinate and had to squat because his knees couldn't support his weight. I worked with him three times and within one session he was already able to lie more comfortably and within three sessions he was able to cock both legs! Now his tail is high, his head carriage is amazing, he looks younger than ever and his vet cannot believe it. And that is just using simple body work and leading exercises through a labyrinth which helped him to use both sides of his brain and therefore think about both sides of his body.'

Sarah Fisher, T-touch practitioner

Using T-touch on your own pets

The nice thing about T-touch is that it is very user-friendly and you cannot do any harm with it. You can learn the basic movements in half an hour. Regular T-touch massage will keep your pet healthy and prevent small problems becoming major complaints. Another good thing about T-touch is that you can work over an injury site, since it is so gentle. It is also a wonderful way of communicating non-verbally with animals and making them feel loved and cared for.

Consulting a T-touch practitioner

Although T-touch is very easy to learn yourself there may be times when the problem is too deep-seated or difficult to handle and you may wish to consult someone who is experienced in treating animals in this way.

With serious problems, always take your pet to the vet first, and ask them to refer you to a T-touch practitioner if this is the treatment you wish for your pet. (See Where to find a T-touch practitioner at the end of the chapter.)

Often a T-touch practitioner will work with your pet a few times and then teach you how to continue the treatment at home and any relevant ground-work exercises that may be helpful.

Any condition that is serious or that does not show signs of improvement quite quickly should be seen by your vet. Never let a pet suffer.

T-touch is a very safe way of working with an animal and it can help in retraining a dog or cat not to behave in a certain way. By opening up new neural pathways, the animal's whole being can be brought back into a state of health and harmony.

How is it done?

Using the middle three fingers of your hand, gently move your hand over the animal's skin in circular movements as if you were drawing a clock face. Start at the six o'clock position and draw a complete circle (clockwise) then continue for another quarter circle. Pause, and then move to another part of the body and draw another circle and a quarter. The main emphasis of this body work is that the movements are random and there should be no pattern to them.

It is an easy method to learn and even children can treat their pets in this way. It also teaches both adults and children to communicate with animals and opens up opportunities for greater respect between the two.

T-touch can be done anywhere since it uses litttle or no equipment which is why it is becoming such a popular method of healing. It is an effective treatment and can work wonders for pets on many different levels.

How many treatments?

How long treatment takes depends on several factors, including how deep-seated the problems is, the age of the animal and the nature of the problem. Normally you would see results within a day or two. The more severe the problem, the longer it is going to take to heal.

For short-term, acute problems treatment usually lasts for 15 minutes, two or three times day. Chronic, long-term problems may need regular daily treatments for several weeks.

Useful information

How to find a T-touch practitioner
UK
Sarah Fisher
South Hill Stables, Radford, Bath BA3 1QQ
Tel: 01761 471182
Fax: 01761 472982

Training in T-touch
UK
Contact Sarah Fisher (above) for details.
T-touch can also be learned from Linda Tellington-Jones' book and video. Viking Press,1992

CHAPTER SIXTEEN

Natural remedies for first-aid use

Natural remedies make great first-aid tools, especially when treating minor, every day things like insect bites or cuts and bruises. In more serious situations, such as road accidents or excessive bleeding, natural remedies offer a therapeutic 'stopgap' until your pet can be seen by a vet.

Always seek veterinary help in emergency situations.

It is well worth getting a first-aid kit together *before* you need it since you never know when you might have to leap into action. The following first-aid kit contains some of the most useful remedies for first-aid use and can be put together simply and inexpensively. Once you acquire more knowledge about other useful remedies you can build up a larger stock of natural healing aids.

First-aid kit for dogs and cats
1. Activated charcoal granules/capsules
These help to delay the absorption of toxins in cases of poisoning. Charcoal also helps remedy digestive upsets and flatulence.

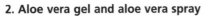

2. Aloe vera gel and aloe vera spray

Aloe vera is a great skin-healer and can be used on cuts, wounds and burns. Aloe vera soothes inflamed skin, protects against infection and speeds the healing process. If you have an aloe vera plant, break off part of the leaf and apply the aloe gel directly to the affected part.

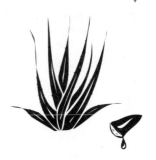

3. Arnica tablets, tincture and cream

Arnica is an essential item in any first-aid kit. It is the first remedy to use for any case of shock and can be used for every kind of injury, wounds, sprains, strains, bruises and swelling. It also helps to stop bleeding. Emotionally, it helps to calm the nerves after an injury. Do not use arnica cream/tincture on broken skin.

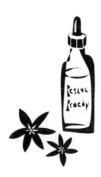

4. Bach flower rescue remedy and rescue remedy cream

Rescue remedy is the first-aid remedy for all emergency situations where there is shock, panic, loss of consciousness or trauma. It can help to alleviate stress and calm an animal down enough so that its mind-body healing processes start working without delay.

5. Calendula cream, calendula tincture

Calendula is used mostly as a topical cream and is a great healing remedy for cuts, burns and bruises. It speeds healing and reduces suppurating and can be used on broken skin.

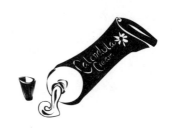

6. Comfrey tincture/ointment/compress

Used as an ointment/tincture on wounds, comfrey is an effective healer once bleeding has stopped. It is especially good for healing broken bones and fractures and can also be applied as a compress.

It can be taken internally as fresh or dried herbs or as capsules to help speed the healing process.

7. Grapefruit-seed extract

Grapefruit-seed extract has been described as *'the world's smallest medicine chest'* and not without good reason. It has proven anti-biotic, anti-fungal, anti-viral, anti-parasitical properties and is an effective disinfectant. It is powerfully effective against a broad spectrum of germs and bacteria but is non-toxic and non-weakening to the immune system – unlike pharmaceutical antibiotics. As a first-aid tool, it can be used externally to clean wounds and prevent infection. Grapefruit-seed extract can be taken internally as well and acts as a natural antibiotic.

Internal use – Add 5–15 drops to food and give 2 or 3 times daily. One capsule = 15 drops.

External use – Dilute 5–10 drops in an eggcup of water to clean cuts and wounds. You can also fill a small spray bottle with grapefruit-seed extract and water for a potent antiseptic spray.

8. Hypericum tablets/tincture/cream

Hypericum is the homoeopathic painkiller. It is particularly good for shooting pain in cases of injury to tails and other extremities. It is also good for cuts and wounds and can be used as a tincture along with calendula to clean wounds. You could also use a combination of calendula and hypericum for painful wounds.

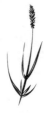

9. Lavender essential oil

This helps to soothe and heal burns and repair scar tissue. Lavender reduces inflammation and encourages healing. Useful for treating wounds and abrasions.

10. Tea tree essential oil, tea tree cream

Tea tree is effective for killing germs and bacteria. It also has cleansing and antiseptic properties. Can be used neat on burns and insect bites, or diluted and used to clean wounds and prevent infection.

11. Witch hazel

Distilled witch hazel used externally helps to reduce inflammation, stop bleeding and ease bruising. Witch hazel is good for cleaning wounds that are still bleeding.

Accidents

A serious accident, such as when an animal is hit by a car, always requires professional help. Once a vet has been called, natural remedies are the next step. While waiting for the vet to arrive, make sure the animal is moved to a safe place, taking care not to change the position it is lying in to prevent further damage. Keep the animal warm and comfortable and talk to it in a soothing voice. Gentle stroking of uninjured areas, particularly the ears, can be very calming and healing for a distressed animal.

The Bach flower rescue remedy can be given immediately to help calm a distressed animal. Also give homoeopathic arnica for shock and injury and to alleviate any bruising. Both these remedies can be given every 10 to 15 minutes in the early stages following an accident. If an animal has lost consciousness and cannot take the remedies, lift up its lip and drop some onto its gums.

Bleeding – excessive/haemorrhage

A small amount of bleeding is quite natural, being nature's way of cleaning out dirt and bacteria, and is not a cause for concern, but excessive bleeding has to be stopped. Severe bleeding can happen if an animal has been in a road traffic accident, got caught on a barbed-wire fence, or been injured in a vicious dog or cat fight.

Immediately call for help and/or take the animal to your nearest vet. In terms of first aid, the best thing to do in cases of excessive bleeding is to put pressure on the wound using whatever padding you have to hand (this may mean using your clothes) until the bleeding stops. Keep a severely haemorrhaging wound raised higher than the heart and try to keep the animal as calm as possible.

Aromatherapy – Once bleeding has stopped lavender oil can be used around the wound area, but not on it. Tea tree oil can be used to clean the wound.

Bach flower remedies – Rescue remedy should be given immediately to calm the animal.

Biochemical tissue salts – Ferr. phos. taken internally or used externally on the wound.

Grapefruit-seed extract – Add a few drops to warm water and use to clean the wound.

Herbs – Goldenseal tincture mixed with water makes a good antiseptic rinse for wounds. A cold compress of witch hazel or rosemary will help to stop bleeding. Aloe vera helps to reduce bleeding and heal wounds and can be used as a spray or as gel applied directly to the wound. Goldenseal and witch hazel can also be used in powder form and made into a paste.

Homoeopathy – Use aconite for shock, followed by arnica to help stem the bleeding given in frequent doses, every 15 minutes at first. Calendula lotion can be used locally to help to heal a wound once bleeding has stopped.

Bruising

Aromatherapy – Lavender oil helps to reduce inflammation and encourage healing.

Bach flower remedies – Use rescue remedy, especially if the animal has also suffered trauma and stress.

Herbs – Witch hazel can be dabbed on bruises with cotton wool to reduce swelling. Also a cold compress of rosemary tea will help reduce bruising and aloe vera gel applied locally also helps to disperse bruising. Alternatively, apply a slice of raw onion to bruises.

Homoeopathy – Arnica tablets can be taken internally. Arnica ointment or tincture can be used topically if the skin is not broken and helps to disperse the bruising. Arnica tincure can be used as a compress (1 teaspoon to 1/2 cup of water). Aconite will help if the animal has suffered stress or trauma as well and it should be given immediately, followed by arnica, every 15 minutes.

Burns and scalds

Cats and dogs often burn or scald themselves by jumping up on a hot cooker or chewing through an electric wire. Any serious burn or scald should always be seen by your vet, but minor ones can be effectively treated at home. One of the best things to do immediately is to submerge the burn in cold water, or if that is not possible use a cold-water compress or an ice pack on the burn. This will help to cool the skin immediately. Honey is very soothing on a burn, and/or use vinegar or a slice of raw onion or potato. Vitamin E can be used directly on burns and scalds – pierce the capsule and gently rub the liquid on the affected area.

Aromatherapy – Rub lavender oil on the burn. This has soothing and antiseptic properties. Tea tree oil is also cleansing and soothing for burns. Geranium helps to heal burned skin.

Bach flower remedies – Rescue remedy.

Biochemical tissue salts – Kali.mur. can be given internally or used topically as a lotion. Use calc. sulph. if the burn/scald is suppurating.

Grapefruit-seed extract – Dilute a few drops in water and use as an anti-septic rinse. You can also use it as a spray if the affected area is too painful to be touched.

Herbs – Aloe vera gel or spray can be applied topically on unbroken skin to accelerate healing. Calendula cream can be used to soothe broken skin.

Homoeopathy – Use arnica for shock and, if there is blistering, urtica for continuous stinging pain, cantharis for pain relief. Once blisters have burst, wash the area with diluted calendula and hypericum tincture 2 or 3 times a day.

Cuts and grazes (also see Wounds)

Minor cuts and grazes are common in pets and can usually be dealt with adequately at home.

Aromatherapy – Tea tree is the best essential oil for cuts and grazes. It has powerful natural antiseptic and anti-bacterial properties. Lavender oil can also be used. Add a few drops to water to clean the wound.

Bach flower remedies – Use rescue remedy given orally. Rescue remedy cream can be used on the cleaned wound.

Grapefruit-seed extract – Use diluted in water as an antiseptic rinse or spray.

Herbs – Aloe vera is a great antiseptic and healer and can be applied topically in gel form or as a spray on a clean wound. You can also use comfrey ointment on a clean wound.

Homoeopathy – Clean the wound with calen-dula or hypericum tinctures. Give arnica tablets if there is any bruising.

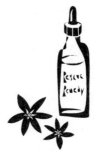

Fractures and broken bones
See musculo-skeletal problems in Chapter 17.

Insect bites and stings
Cats and dogs often chase insects and sometimes end up getting stung. Both bites and stings can penetrate the skin and cause swelling, redness and even infection. Always clean the wound before treatment.

Aromatherapy – Lavender oil is soothing and helps to ease stinging and burning sensations. Geranium or tea tree oils help to relieve pain and ease itching.

Bach flower remedies – Give rescue remedy orally. Rescue remedy cream can be used topically on bites and stings.

Biochemical tissue salts – Nat. mur. can be applied externally to the wound in the form of a paste.

Grapefruit-seed extract – Use undiluted on the bite or sting to prevent infection. If the area is very sensitive, use it diluted in water. Grapefruit-seed extract can also be used as a spray.

Herbs – Marigold ointment can help to reduce swelling. For wasp or bee stings, remove the sting with tweezers and dab some vinegar on the wound and then place a slice of fresh onion over it. A drop of nettle extract (urtica) can ease stings. Aloe vera gel/spray is soothing and cooling and the spray can be used as an insect repellant.

Homoeopathy – Apis mel. is soothing for swollen and red stings, such as wasp stings., Hypericum for horsefly bites. You can use hypericum or hypercal tinctures to clean bite wounds. Calendula ointment can also be applied to bites.

Poisoning
Cats and dogs can be poisoned by all sorts of things including garden chemicals, slug pellets, household chemicals and medicines. Poisoning can also be the result of an evening's garbage raiding! and the most obvious symptoms are vomiting and diarrhoea. Always call your vet if you suspect poisoning since treatment will vary depending on what the animal has swallowed. It may not always be the best thing to make them sick so always err on the safe side and wait for the vet. If possible keep some of the suspected poison (including vomit or diarrhoea) to help identify what it was that they ate.

In terms of first aid, one of the best things to do is to delay the absorption of the poison using activated charcoal granules/capsules. Mix about 5 heaped teaspoons in a cup of water (or empty out the contents of capsules). Give this mixture to your pet, using 1/4 to a full cupful depending on their size. Use a syringe if necessary.

Bach flower remedies – Give rescue remedy immediately. Use crab apple for cleansing, olive for exhausted and sick animals.

Grapefruit-seed extract – In cases of food poisoning, add 5–15 drops to an eggcup of water and try to get your pet to drink it. It can sometimes be easier to fill a syringe and carefully put the liquid directly into their mouth or if they will eat, then add it to something tasty. Give 2 or 3 times a day.

Herbs – Milk thistle given afterwards will help to repair any liver damage as a result of the poison. Aloe vera juice is also a good all-round intestinal detoxifier. Cat's claw helps to boost the immune system.

Homoeopathy – Give aconite for shock associated with poisoning, nux vomica for poisoning by plants or foods and arsenic for associated pain and restlessness, acute vomiting or diarrhoea. The animal may want to drink little and often.

Shock/trauma/loss of consciousness

Shock and trauma are very common after an accident and an animal will display symptoms of rapid breathing, whitened gums and might also fall unconscious. The first thing to do is to call the vet or take them there. In terms of first aid, there is much you can do until professional help arrives.

Aromatherapy – Put a few drops of lavender or peppermint oil on a handkerchief and hold this under your pet's nose. You can also use diluted lavender to massage into their ears. There is a shock point at the tip of the ear which, when massaged, will help to calm an animal.

Bach flower remedies – Rescue remedy is a wonderful remedy for all cases of shock. If the animal is unconscious, lift the flap of their mouth and drop some rescue remedy in, or rub some drops into the fur behind their ears. Star of Bethlehem is also good for trauma or injury.

Biochemical tissue salts – Give nat. sulph. Place the tablets in the mouth of an unconscious animal, where they will quickly dissolve.

Homoeopathy – Aconite is the first remedy to use in all cases of shock, followed by arnica. Place the remedies in the mouth of an unconscious animal where it will dissolve quickly. They can be given every 15 minutes if necessary.

Sprains and strains
See musculo-skeletal problems in Chapter 17.

Sunstroke/overheating
The most likely cause of this is when a pet is left in a hot car – they can even fall unconscious. Always park your car in the shade and leave a window or sunroof fully open if leaving an animal for any length of time. It only takes a short while for an animal to overheat. Make sure plenty of fresh water is also available to them.

Sunstroke and overheating can be fatal, so always call your vet. The next step is to get the animal into the shade and soak them with cool water. If possible use an ice pack around their head to cool the brain and, if they are conscious, see if they will drink some water.

Bach flower remedies – Rescue remedy is the emergency remedy.

Homoeopathy – Use aconite to relieve shock and early effects of heat-stroke. Give belladonna if there is also great thirst.

Wounds (also see cuts and grazes and bleeding)
Dogs and cats can be wounded in all sorts of ways, including traffic accidents and fights. Serious wounds, like puncture wounds, always need veterinary attention, but many minor wounds such as scratches, or getting their tail caught in a door, can often be treated at home. The healing of post-operative wounds can also be greatly helped by natural remedies.

Aromatherapy – Lavender oil is cleansing and antiseptic and can be used near the wound but not on it. Tea tree oil can be used on wounds and is a powerful antiseptic.

Bach flowers remedies – Use rescue remedy taken orally or used topically as cream. Give star of Bethlehem for trauma and injury.

Biochemical tissue salts – Use ferr. phos. externally and internally, calc. sulph. for sup-purating wounds.

Grapefruit-seed extract – Use diluted to clean the wound and prevent infection. Add 12 drops to an eggcup of water.

Herbs – Aloe vera is a natural antiseptic and can be used to clean the wound. Aloe vera gel rubbed on afterwards reduces bruising and aids healing of damaged tissue. A poultice of slippery elm draws out pus or any foreign bodies from the wound.

Homoeopathy – Arnica helps prevent bruising, stop bleeding and accelerate the healing of damaged tissue. Use ledum for wounds if there is a risk of tetanus and hypericum for shooting pains often associated with tail injuries. Calendula lotion has remarkable healing properties and can be used directly on wounds. Use hypericum ointment when there are shooting pains. Calendula and hypericum tinctures can be used to clean a wound. Goldenseal tincture also makes a good antiseptic rinse.

Vitamins – Vitamin E used topically helps to promote skin healing.

CHAPTER SEVENTEEN

Specific ailments and treatments

This chapter lists a number of common complaints and conditions that can be helped by natural treatments and remedies. Many of the remedies can be used safely and effectively at home, but if your pet has a serious condition you should seek veterinary advice as well.

In the same way as you would assess your own health or a child's health, it is a matter of using your common sense and deciding whether your pet can be effectively treated at home or whether you need to take it to the vet. More and more vets are incorporating complementary treatments into their practice, but if your own vet does not practise complementary medicine, then ask them to refer you to an holistic vet. Many vets are also happy to refer you to a chiropractor, healer or some other similarly qualified practitioner who treats animals, as long as they are kept up to date with the course of treatment your pet is receiving. Be firm about getting the treatment you want for your pet.

When using natural remedies yourself or seeking professional help for your pet, make sure you understand how the treatments and remedies work and know what you can realistically expect. When used correctly, natural remedies make wonderful healing tools and, the more you can learn about natural medicine, the more you can help your pet to stay healthy and happy. Preventing illness with a good diet and treating simple things yourself allows you to take a more active and positive role in your pet's health.

Nothing can take the place of preventative medicine, which is why a natural diet and supplement programme is vitally important and will enhance the effects of every other treatment. A complete recovery or a return to optimum health can only happen when your pet is on a good diet, since an inadequate diet may have been the very thing that caused their illness in the first place!

When using the remedies at home, choose one type of treatment at a time. As mentioned earlier, more is not better and different remedies can interfere with each other. If you choose to use herbs, for example, then pick one or two from the recommended list and let them have a chance to work before trying another herb or another remedy. With homoeopathy, use the remedy that most fits the symptoms and only use another if it does not bring about an improvement. In the same way, it is best to use one treatment type at a time and not book your pet an appointment with a chiropractor, a healer and a homoeopath all in the same week! It is also important to read the chapter on your chosen remedy for information on how to use the remedies and what doses to give. Where relevant, some of the chapters include details of putting together a basic medicine chest for that particular remedy. The more you understand about natural medicine and how to use it, the more responsible you can be for your pet's health.

Remember too that natural remedies work more gently and more slowly than fast-acting, modern drugs, so be patient. There may be times when drugs are the first choice, and natural treatments can be used afterwards to support the recovery process.

The following chart is a quick reference guide to the most suitable treatments and remedies for each complaint and condition. Although natural medicine, when used holistically, will have a positive effect on all disease (be it physical, emotional, mental or spiritual), some treatments can be more effective than others depending on specific complaints.

	Diet and Supplements	Acupuncture	Aroma-therapy	Biochemical Tissue Salts	Chiropractic	Flower Essences	Healing	Herbs	Homoeo-opathy	T-touch
Behavioural Problems	2	1	2	1	0	3	3	2	2	3
Cancer	3	2	1	1	0	1	3	3	2	1
Cardiovascular System	3	2	1	2	1	1	2	2	2	1
Digestive System	3	2	2	2	1	1	3	3	3	1
Ear Problems	2	1	3	1	0	1	1	3	3	0
Eye Problems	2	3	1	1	0	1	2	3	3	0
Immune System	3	3	2	2	1	2	3	3	3	1
Kidney & Urinary	3	2	2	2	1	1	2	3	2	1
Muscle & Joint Problems	3	3	2	2	3	1	2	2	2	3
Operations	3	3	2	1	1	2	3	2	2	1
Parasites	3	1	1	1	0	1	1	2	2	0
Pregnancy	3	2	3	1	2	2	1	3	2	1
Respiratory System	3	3	2	1	1	1	2	2	3	1
Skin & Coat	3	2	2	1	1	2	2	3	3	1
Spaying and Neutering	2	2			0	3	3	2	2	3
Pain Relief	1	3	2	1	2	1	3	1	2	2

KEY
0 – least appropriate treatment in this case
1 – will have positive results, but less effective than other treatments in this case
2 – effective treatment
3 – very effective, first choice of treatment
■ – suitable to use at home

BEHAVIOURAL PROBLEMS

Behavioural problems in pets can be caused by a number of things and in many cases there are underlying emotional or mental problems that need to be addressed. Flower remedies and healing are particularly good treatments for behavioural problems and it is important to read Chapters 11 and 12 to get a fuller understanding of emotional and mental problems in pets and how they can be helped.

Many of the problems displayed by our pets bear a close resemblance to our own behavioural patterns. Pets often mirror what is going on for us mentally and emotionally. It is therefore really important to look at the stresses around the home and to address these in order to bring about a complete change. Pets whose owners are going through a divorce, for example, may display behavioural problems, just like children often do. When treating pets with behavioural problems, very often the owner will also need to take the same remedy.

Many behavioural problems stem back to negative experiences in an animal's early life and these too can be treated with natural remedies.

Causes of behavioural problems are many and varied and include: poor breeding (viciousness, repetitive habits, nervous-system imbalances), poor nutrition, frequent or multiple vaccinations, inadequate exercise, lack of stimulation and attention, too much attention, past abuse, current stress, excessive attachment to a pet, inappropriate expectations of a pet and being treated like a human being, not an animal!

Because of its holistic nature, natural medicine has a lot to offer animals with behavioural problems. Suitable treatments include acupuncture, aromatherapy, biochemical tissue salts, diet and supplements, flower remedies, healing, herbs, homoeopathy and T-touch.

Abused animals

See Aggression and biting, and Nervousness, anxiety and fear in the following pages.

Aggression and biting

Aggression in the right circumstances is entirely healthy and normal, but inappropriate aggression is not. A dog who bites the postman or a cat that scratches visitors for no reason makes an unpredictable and unsociable pet, and in some cases a dangerous one. Some breeds are more aggressive than others, but mostly there are underlying reasons for aggressive behaviour, such as fear, bad breeding, jealousy, past abuse, hyperactivity, stress, vaccine damage, allergies, pain, and illness. Aggressive behaviour is often a symptom of a deeper underlying emotional or mental problem and once this is healed, inappropriate aggression will usually disappear.

Diet – A natural preservative-free or allergy diet is an essential first step towards curing behavioural problems which may be caused by an intolerance to particular foods or food additives. Oats have a calming effect and can be made into a porridge. Anti-stress supplements include raw honey, brewer's yeast (or a B complex vitamin), vitamin C, vitamin E and zinc. You can also give bone-meal and a good-quality, multi-mineral and vitamin formula (see Chapters 4 and 5 for details).

Aromatherapy – Touch is an important element in healing disturbed animals and a massage can be very relaxing and calming for them. Sandalwood, ylang ylang and lavender oils can be used for massage or used in a diffuser or burner.

Bach flower remedies – Use chicory for possessiveness, water violet for cats and dogs with a wild ancestry, holly for jealousy and animals quick to anger with a tendency to bite, impatiens for irritability, cherry plum for animals who lose control in aggressive situations and beech for intolerance.

Herbs – The most commonly used herbs for soothing and calming are chamomile, scullcap and valerian.

Homoeopathy – Use belladonna for anger and a tendency to bite, nux vomica for irritability and arsenicum for anger and attacks of panic.

Bad habits

Also see Spraying (cats), Aggression and biting, and Nervousness, anxiety and fear in this section.

Bach flower remedies – Chestnut bud is a good remedy for animals with bad habits to break, such as chewing shoes or furniture, or raiding the rubbish bin.

Barking/mewing (excessive)

See Hyperactivity, Bad habits in this section.

Depression

Also see Grief, pining and bereavement, below.

Bach flower remedies – Use mustard for depression.

Eating own faeces or other animal's faeces

See Appetite problems and Digestive problems in this chapter, and Bad habits, above.

Grief, pining and bereavement

Just like us, animals get attached to places and people and their loss can cause feelings of depression, pain and grief. If a pet's owner dies an animal can become overwhelmed by grief, and many of these animals end up in rescue centres – which further adds to their stress. There are lots of stories about the incredible bonding that can happen between a human being and an animal, and if you have been lucky enough to experience its strength you can appreciate just how emotionally developed animals are. Helping a pet overcome grief takes time, patience and love.

Diet – A good-quality natural diet is very important during stressful times, and it helps to boost an animal's immune system. See Stress, in this section, for helpful supplements. Also see Chapters 4 and 5 for diet and supplement recommendations.

Aromatherapy – Massage and touch are very therapeutic for depressed or grief-stricken animals. They need more love and attention at this time and will greatly benefit from regular, relaxing massages. Use neroli for improved mood, sweet marjoram and lavender to help with sleep, basil and sweet marjoram for depression.

Bach flower remedies – Star of Bethlehem for emotional trauma, past or present, and is especially helpful for animals in rescue centres. Use honeysuckle for grief or homesickness, for an animal that has lost its mate or owner, or when in boarding kennels. Mustard for depression and mood swings, pine for rejected animals, walnut to help pets adapt to change, crab apple to release negative emotions from the past (eg past abuse), and red chestnut for worrying, pining animals waiting for their owner to come home.

Herbs – Use chamomile, scullcap and valerian to calm and reduce stress.

Homoeopathy – Use ignatia for bereavement, pining, grief and homesickness.

Hyperactivity

Hyperactivity in pets includes things like excessive barking or mewing, constantly jumping up and seeking attention, rarely relaxing, becomes easily excited, irritability, biting and scratching, nervy and anxious, and being oversexed or difficult to train.

Some cases can be put down to bad breeding, allergies, boredom, stress, frequent or multiple vaccination, insecurity, lack of stimulation, inadequate exercise, lack of routine, excess protein, lack of love and attention. Although some breeds are naturally highly strung, most hyperactivity is rooted in underlying emotional or mental problems, inadequate feeding, stress around the home, and allergies.

Diet – Very often hyperactivity in pets is related to an intolerance to certain foods and food additives. Changing to a natural preservative-free diet is sometimes enough on its own to cure the problem. Oats have a calming effect and can be used as a porridge. Specific supplements for hyperactivity include brewer's yeast (or vitamin-B complex), vegetable and fish oils, bone-meal, vitamin C. Also see Stress, in this section, and Chapters 4 and 5 for more details.

Aromatherapy – Massage can be very relaxing for restless, hyperactive pets. Calming oils include lavender, sweet marjoram, basil and chamomile. They can also be used in a diffuser or burner.

Bach flower remedies – Use rock rose for panic attacks, vervain for highly strung, hyperactive animals.

Biochemical tissue salts – Kali. phos. is a good nerve tonic.

Herbs – Use oat straw tincture, scullcap and valerian for calming. Aloe vera and kelp are useful detoxifiers when allergies are suspected.

Homoeopathy – Use scutellaria (scullcap) for highly strung, often destructive pets, belladonna for excitable, aggressive pets.

Moving home

Also see Grief, pining and bereavement in this section.

Bach flower remedies – Walnut helps an animal adapt to change. Scleranthus eases travel sickness.

Homoeopathy – Ignatia helps with accepting new surroundings.

Nervousness, anxiety, fear

A nervous, anxious animal is often one that has had a bad experience earlier in its life, such as an accident, abuse, abandonment, frequent change of owner or neglect. Pets can be nervy and highly strung all the time or scared of specific things like thunderstorms, small children, vacuum cleaners and hair dryers. A nervous animal is often unpredictable and may bite or scratch without good reason.

Other causes of nervous behaviour include allergies to foods or chemicals, and physical illness.

Natural remedies can help to calm a nervous animal and heal emotional or mental stress that is causing their behavioural problems. With behavioural problems it is always a good idea to evaluate the stress in the home, since your pet may be reacting to its emotional environment. T-touch and healing are effective treatments in addition to those listed below.

Diet – Behavioural problems are often related to food intolerances, so changing your pet's food to a natural preservative-free or allergy diet is essential. Oats added to the diet have a soothing and calming effect. Certain supplements are helpful in combating stress and can be included in the diet eg vitamins C, E, A, and D, B complex, zinc, calcium and magnesium. Use a good-quality, multi-vitamin and mineral supplement containing these or add them individually to the diet. See Chapters 4 and 5 for details.

Aromatherapy – Massage is relaxing and comforting for anxious pets. Use a combination of the following oils: chamomile, neroli, lavender and sweet marjoram.

Bach flower remedies – Use aspen for anxiety and apprehension, but not specific fears. For the kind of animal that always seems a little troubled or anxious, for no apparent reason, never quite settled or content. Use mimulus for specific fears like a fear of thunderstorms, rock rose for terror, extreme fright, panic, rescue remedy for sudden fear or shock, star of Bethlehem for past traumas not fully recovered from.

Biochemical tissue salts – Kali. phos. is a good nerve tonic.

Herbs – Chamomile, scullcap and valerian are all calming herbs.

Homoeopathy – Use aconite to minimise fear before or after a frightening experience such as fireworks or thunderstorms. Give gelsemium when rigid with fear, phosphorus for fear of sudden noises and argent nit. for restless, anxious pets.

Oversexed
See Hyperactivity in this section.

Spraying (cats) – inappropriately

Usually some kind of stress is at the root of inappropriate spraying, when cats suddenly begin marking the house with urine. Things like a new arrival to the household, moving home or shock can trigger stress-related problems. Natural treatments and remedies work very well for problems like these. Follow the guidelines for stress and nervousness or use the following remedies.

Aromatherapy – Spray areas of the house that your cat sprays with natural repellent aromas like lemon oil, geranium and eucalyptus. They will soon get the message! Dilute a few drops of oil in a base of vodka and water and use as a repellent spray.

Bach flower remedies – Use willow for resentment and anger, chestnut bud for bad habits.

Stress

Stress is something we all seem to suffer from these days, and so do our pets. Many pets do not live a natural life and are fed on what amounts to 'convenience' food for animals. Often dogs get left alone for hours on end in a city flat, and some cats never get outside their entire lives. All of these things are highly stressful and are not a good recipe for mental or emotional health, and eventually animals display behavioural problems as a result.

Our pets also pick up our stress and mirror our moods. It is therefore a good idea to treat owners and pets with the same remedies! Stress-related diseases are on the increase, and there is a lot you can do to help reduce your own and your pet's stress levels.

Diet – A natural preservative-free diet and supplement programme will enhance your pet's health and help them to cope with stress. Specific supplements for stress include brewer's yeast (or a B complex), vitamins C and E, calcium, magnesium, zinc, raw honey, royal jelly and oats (see Chapters 4 and 5.

Herbs – Siberian ginseng, liquorice and gota kola help the body cope with stress. Chamomile, oat straw, scullcap and valerian are all calming. Massage, healing and T-touch are also excellent for stressed pets. Also see Nervousness, anxiety and fear.

CANCER

Cancerous tissue can grow literally anywhere in or on the body. Sometimes the cancer is obvious, such as a skin tumour, but other times it is not, as in the case with liver cancer. There are many causes of cancer in cats and dogs, including pollution, stress, electrical emissions (televisions, mains supply etc), frequent or multiple vaccinations, inadequate diet, chemical additives, colourings and preservatives, unnatural residues in food from agricultural chemicals. Cats and dogs are affected by pollution in the environment, food and water just as we are, and this damages their immune system. If the immune system is damaged, the body's natural ability to fight cancerous cells is impaired.

Natural remedies and treatments can help to alleviate symptoms and boost the immune system to fight against cancer. (Also see Immune system in this chapter.) The emphasis is always on prevention, so that your pet is not exposed to excess pollutants in their food, water or environment in the first place. If an animal can be kept in peak health, its immune system will remain strong and it will be more resistant to cancer-causing agents. A poor diet is a major factor in cancer, whereas a natural diet boosts the animal's own powers of self-healing and resistance to disease. It is also worth rethinking vaccinating your pet (see Chapter 6). Also, eliminate any possible toxins, such as commercial flea collars, worming tablets, flea powder, insecticides, room deodorisers, strong chemical cleaners and tobacco smoke.

Suitable treatments include acupuncture, aromatherapy, diet and supplements, flower essences, healing, herbs, homoeopathy.

Before treating your pet at home, always read the relevant chapters on the treatments and remedies you are planning to use for information of dosage, and how each of the treatments work. In the case of serious disease, initially you may need to combine conventional drugs with natural remedies.

Diet – A natural preservative-free diet is the most important factor in the prevention and treatment of cancer. Use organic foods where possible, especially if your pet already has cancer, to make sure the diet is as pollutant-free as possible. Use filtered or bottled water, not tap water. Helpful foods in the diet include dried apricots, carrots, broccoli, potatoes, watercress, beetroot, cabbage, tomato, turnip and garlic. Raw sweetbreads (thymus) and organic liver are also 'positive' foods. Apple cider vinegar added to food or water helps to keep the internal acid/alkaline balance right, which is important in preventing and arresting the spread of cancer. More wonderful additions to the diet are freshly made juices, especially carrot juice and green juices, such as cabbage, pepper and lettuce. Also give B-complex vitamins, high doses of vitamin C (double the normal dose), vitamin A (1000–3,000iu), vitamin E (200–600iu), royal jelly, kelp and alfalfa or other green food such as barley grass/spirulina. Oats are strengthening. In addition, give fish oil, evening primrose oil and vegetable oils, along with a good-quality, multi-mineral and vitamin complex, digestive enzymes and probiotics. Acorn Supplements Ltd (UK) make a great product called Immune Plus which includes herbs, probiotics, vitamins, minerals and trace elements, and Pet Plus, a combined probiotic and digestive enzyme formula (see Chapter 5).

Aromatherapy – Ylang ylang and rosemary are revitalising and can be burned in a diffuser or massaged into your pet's skin.

Herbs – Mistletoe has anti-tumour properties. Immune-strengthening herbs include garlic, cat's claw, astragalus and echinacea. Milk thistle strengthens and repairs the liver. Oat tincture is strengthening. Aloe vera and liquid chlorophyll help to nourish and detoxify the system. Acorn Supplements Ltd (UK) supply Flor.Essence a herbal formula with remarkable cleansing and healing properties found to be helpful in cancer treatment.

Homoeopathy – Use hydrastis in early cases of cancer. Arsen. alb. relieves pain. Use thuja for warty tumours. Viscum. alb. is beneficial in most cases of cancer.

CARDIOVASCULAR SYSTEM

The cardiovascular system includes the heart and blood and the circulatory system. Heart and circulation problems are relatively common in older pets and include things like a weak heart muscle, high blood pressure, thickening of the heart muscle, heart failure, an irregular pulse and anaemia.

Some of the commonest causes of heart problems are obesity, a high-stress lifestyle, hereditary factors, poor nutrition, pollution, and toxic chemicals in food and water.

Signs to look out for if you suspect your pet has heart trouble are laboured breathing, a persistent dry cough, coughing after exercise or during the night, fluid retention in the legs and abdomen and extreme nervousness. There may be a bluish look to the tongue and gums.

Any heart or circulation problems should always be checked out by your vet, since poor circulation can ultimately affect other organs like the liver and kidneys.

Heart disease can be prevented by giving your pet a healthy, low-stress lifestyle, nutritious food and regular exercise. Natural treatments and remedies can help treat heart and circulation problems and work well as a preventative measure. Suitable treatments include acupuncture, aromatherapy, biochemical tissue salts, chiropractic, diet and food supplements, flower essences, healing, herbs, homoeopathy, T-touch. Before treating your pet at home read the relevant chapters for information on treatment, remedies, dosage, suppliers etc.

Heart and circulation problems

Diet – Pets fed on natural diets rarely get heart disease. Processed foods and inadequate diet are two of the biggest contributory factors, so change your pet's diet to one that is natural and preservative-free. Sugar (including honey) and salt should be entirely omitted. Add plenty of vegetables to the daily diet and some cooked whole grains for dogs. Garlic lowers blood pressure and cholesterol. Watercress is a good circulation tonic. Use only filtered or bottled water. Apple cider vinegar adds potassium. For overweight dogs and cats see Weight problems and overweight/obesity in this chapter. Useful supplements include royal jelly, magnesium, calcium, B complex, vitamin C, vitamin E (not for very weak hearts until stabilised), cod-liver oil, evening primrose oil, lecithin and digestive enzymes. Green super-foods add extra nutrients and seaweed (kelp) is also an excellent supplement for keeping the blood and circulation healthy – every mineral normally found in healthy blood is found in seaweed. Kelp also lowers high blood pressure (see Chapters 4 and 5 for details).

Exercise – Moderate, regular exercise is good for the heart and circulation.

Aromatherapy – Massage with lavender, clary sage, ylang ylang, mint and ginger.

Bach flower remedies – Use oak for strengthening very weak animals, impatiens for nervousness, and hornbeam for weak, fatigued animals.

Biochemical tissue salts – Use kali. phos. if the problem is due to nervous excitement. Calc. flour. restores strength to the heart muscle.

Herbs – Hawthorn berry tincture is a heart-muscle repairer and general heart tonic. Dandelion, parsley, watercress are mildly diuretic. Use ginger to stimulate circulation and scullcap to calm. Ginkgo Biloba improves vascular flow and improves oxygen delivery to the tissues.

Homoeopathy – Crataegus (hawthorn berries) are the main remedy for heart problems with breathing difficulty, irregular/weak pulse, high blood pressure, fluid retention, weak heart, irritability and nervousness.

Anaemia

Anaemia is a lack of red blood corpuscles in the blood. It is the red blood corpuscles that carry oxygen round the body to the organs and tissues and are therefore vital to life. Causes of anaemia include blood loss from wounds, parasites (fleas and worms), underproduction of red blood corpuscles, internal bleeding and poisons eg rat poison, and toxic metals like lead. Underproduction of red blood corpuscles can be caused by iron deficiency, inadequate diet, viruses, and kidney disease.

Signs and symptoms of anaemia include sluggishness, lack of energy and vitality, pale gums and pale membranes around the inner rim of the eyelid, weight loss, lack of appetite and depression. Always take your pet to your vet for a diagnosis in case there is a serious underlying problem.

Diet – Change to a natural preservative-free diet as recommended in Chapter 4. Increase the amount of iron-rich foods such as red meat, liver, eggs, lentils, green-leaf vegetables, spinach, watercress, blackstrap molasses, and red foods – beetroot, black grapes, red pepper and apricots. Prunes, figs and raisins are also 'positive' foods for anaemia. Digestive enzymes will help with the absorption of nutrients. Kelp and green super-foods add valuable extra nutrients. Use a good-quality multi-vitamin and mineral complex which includes vitamin C, B complex, vitamin B12, folic acid, (or give brewer's yeast for the B group of vitamins), copper, iron, calcium, magnesium. (Vitamin C and copper help the absorption of iron.) (See Chapters 4 and 5.)

Aromatherapy – Wild marjoram will help to invigorate tired, exhausted animals.

Bach flower remedies – Use olive for exhaustion or an ill animal, hornbeam to strengthen.

Biochemical tissue salts – Use ferr. phos., calc. phos.

Herbs – Use alfalfa, dandelion, nettle and parsley. Nettle and parsley in particular supply plenty of iron and vitamin C.

Homoeopathy – Use ferrum met., if inadequate nutrition is a factor, phosphorus for persistent bleeding leading to anaemia, china after blood loss leading to weakness, nux vomica after blood loss with irritability and silicea for underlying constitutional factors.

DIGESTIVE PROBLEMS

The digestive system starts in the mouth and ends at the anus and includes the stomach, intestines, liver, kidneys and pancreas. This section covers many of the more common problems relating to the whole digestive process including dental disease, weight problems, colic, colitis, liver, kidney and pancreatic disease, constipation and diarrhoea, malabsorption, bad breath, flatulence, allergies, and travel sickness. The single most important treatment for digestive problems is a good diet; therefore it is essential to read Chapters 4 and 5 if treating any of the following complaints.

Suitable treatments include acupuncture, aromatherapy, biochemical tissue salts, diet, food supplements, flower essences, healing, herbs, homoeopathy. Before treating your pet at home, read the relevant chapters for information on treatment, remedies, dosage and suppliers etc.

Allergies

Allergies or food sensitivities are on the increase both in humans and in pets, and many people would say it is because our food and environment are becoming increasingly polluted and our lifestyles more stressed and unhealthy – this goes for our pets too! Multiple or frequent vaccination is also thought to be a major factor in immune-related diseases.

An allergic reaction is an adverse response by the immune system to something that is normally harmless to the body, such as wheat, beef or plant pollen. Reactions can range from sneezing and watery eyes to diarrhoea and skin rashes. Contributing factors are a poorly functioning digestive system, an overburdened or weakened immune system, weakened liver function due to excess toxins and stress.

The most common trigger foods are milk, beef, pork, chicken, wheat gluten, soya, food additives, grasses, pollens, moulds, house dust, house dust mites, fleas, household chemicals and washing powder. Reactions can be many and varied including: skin problems, itching, scratching, inflamed ears, digestive upsets, diarrhoea, constipation, urinary tract infections, vomiting, hair loss, rashes, hyperactivity and other behavioural disturbances.

There is a lot that can be done with natural treatments, although it can take time and effort. (Also see Skin and coat, Fleas, Immune system in this chapter and other relevant ailments, such as Runny nose, Diarrhoea, Eczema and dermatitis also in this chapter.)

Diet – About a third of allergies are thought to be caused by food therefore fasting and a change of diet is the best way to start (see Chapter 4). By reducing your pet's diet to a few foods (preferably organic) and then gradually introducing more foods, the 'triggers' can usually be spotted and subsequently avoided. Commercially made pet food contains many potential allergens, such as beef, wheat, chemicals, colourings, preservatives, flavourings and agricultural chemical residues. Drinking water needs to be filtered, or use bottled spring water, but not tap water. As supplements, give digestive enzymes, probiotics and a good-quality, multi-mineral and vitamin complex. Also give additional vitamin C (500–5,000mg daily) and a non-yeast source of vitamin-B complex (see Chapters 4 and 5).

Environment – Eliminate any possible environmental triggers such as commercial flea collars, flea powder, insecticides, room deodorisers, strong chemical cleaners and tobacco smoke.

Bach flower remedies – Use rescue remedy for sudden, uncomfortable reactions. Crab apple for cleansing.

Herbs – Cat's claw, garlic, astragalus and echinacea help support the immune system. Use aloe vera and liquid chlorophyll for detoxification and healing the gut. Chamomile will help soothe an allergic response. Use milk thistle (silymarin) and dandelion to support the liver.

Homoeopathy – Various remedies can be used to treat the allergy symptoms eg runny nose, skin rash etc (see specific symptoms). Seek the advice of a homoeopathic vet for holistic treatment. For people allergic to cat or dog fur, Ainsworths (UK) make remedies from pet hairs which can reduce the sensitivity and severity of attack (see Chapter 14).

Appetite problems

Appetite problems include lack of appetite, excessive appetite or depraved appetite (eg eating own faeces).

Loss of appetite

(See also Underweight in this section.) This is usually a sign of illness and animals will naturally fast when they are feeling unwell. During a fast, energy is directed away from digestion, towards healing. Once they begin to feel better they will soon want to eat again. If the problem does not resolve itself fairly quickly, then take your pet to the vet for a thorough examination. Loss of appetite can be a sign of a range of illnesses from worms or fur balls to diabetes and pancreatic disease.

Dogs usually have good appetites, but cats can develop finicky eating to the extent that they will only eat a few select foods. Try not to let this happen. It is always best to keep a wide range of foods in your pet's diet and if they don't eat it at one meal, take the food away and dish it up at the next. A healthy cat will eventually eat when it gets hungry enough! Most pets that are finicky eaters are given snacks between meals, or their dish is left around with food in it between meals. This encourages fussy eaters. Cats are also prone to becoming anorexic, especially if they have had a trauma, an operation or just feel that their life is over and stop eating. Bach flower remedies can help when emotional reasons lie behind appetite loss. To encourage eating try 'lacing' their food with tempting flavours and ingredients until they get back to normal eating again.

Diet – Change to a natural preservative-free diet which can be 'laced' with tasty bites to encourage eating. Feed small meals at a time and take the food away if your pet does not eat it within half an hour. As a supplement, give a good-quality, multi-mineral and vitamin complex. Add extra zinc (5–15mg). Zinc deficiency is strongly indicated in anorexia and a lack of taste or smell which may be the underlying causes of poor appetite.

Bach flower remedies – Loss of appetite is often linked to emotional factors – refer to Chapter 11 for appropriate remedies.

Herbs – Herbs that stimulate appetite include peppermint, watercress and chamomile.

Homoeopathy – Use arsen. alb. for pets that seem interested in eating but then change their mind. Give carbo. veg. for loss of appetite due to digestive upsets.

Excessive or depraved appetite

An excessive or depraved appetite is usually a sign that the animal is not getting a good-quality nutritious diet or that it is not absorbing nutrients properly because its digestion is at fault. Sometimes pets will eat their own or other animal's faeces in an attempt to get nutrients. Other causes of excessive or depraved appetite include intestinal worms, heart disease, pancreatic or liver disease.

Diet – This is the most important thing to address. First change their diet to a natural preservative-free diet since allergy or incorrect diet may be the underlying cause. If malabsorption is the problem, the digestive process can be helped by adding digestive enzymes to their food. Probiotics help to get the right intestinal environment for optimum absorption of nutrients. A toxic intestinal system can also impede nutrient absorption, therefore psyllium husks added to food will help to clean out the bowel and remove toxins.

Herbs – Aloe vera juice is rich in easily absorbed nutrients and can be added to food. Also alfalfa which can be added to food or use liquid chlorophyll.

Homoeopathy – Use calc. carb. for depraved appetite in fat animals, calc. phos. for thin animals. Also see Weight problems and Parasites.

Bad breath

The most common cause of bad breath is gum disease, so it is worth checking this out first (see also Teeth and gums). Other causes of bad breath include digestive problems, liver and kidney problems or worms (see also Parasites).

Colic

Colic is a gripping, spasmodic pain in the animal's abdomen which can either come in intervals or happen so regularly that it seems like one continuous spasm. Symptoms of colic include obvious discomfort, gurgling noises in the stomach, flatulence, panting, distress, whining or mewing with pain. The most common causes are inadequate diet, impaired digestion and allergies.

Diet – Colic is a sign that the digestive system is not working properly or that the diet is at fault. A change of diet to one that is natural and preservative-free is essential. You may also need to add digestive enzymes to your pet's food in the initial stages of healing and probiotics (friendly gut bacteria). Alfalfa helps with the assimilation of nutrients. Watercress aids digestion. (See also Colitis, Flatulence and Parasites). Follow the dietary guidelines in Chapters 4 and 5.

Aromatherapy – Chamomile, peppermint and caraway oils can be massaged into the abdomen.

Bach flower remedies – Use crab apple for cleansing.

Biochemical tissue salts – Use mag. phos. with cramps, combination E for colic pains, indigestion and flatulence.

Herbs – Aloe vera has a soothing effect on the digestive system. Also slippery elm, goldenseal, ginger, chamomile and peppermint. Parsley and fenugreek are digestive tonics. Liquorice is anti-inflammatory and soothing.

Homoeopathy – Use nux vomica for chronic cases, colocynthis for acute cases where the pain comes in waves.

Colitis

Colitis is an inflammation of the colon (large intestine) and can be acute (short-term) or chronic (long-term). Signs that your pet is suffering from colitis include diarrhoea or constipation, frequent bowel movements, straining, blood and/or mucus in the stools, abdominal pain and weight loss. There seems to be a wide range of causes of colitis but a few of the more common ones are allergies, stress, parasites, and inadequate diet.

Diet – Diet is the most important factor in treating digestive problems and although colitis may be difficult to cure completely, it can be kept well under control with dietary measures. A high fibre diet is very important for both dogs and cats and one of the main ingredients of the diet should be cooked brown rice. Other helpful foods include live yoghurt, oats, carrots, apples and cabbage. If your pet has colitis you should also suspect allergies, especially to wheat gluten. A diet based on lamb, chicken or turkey and rice is usually well tolerated. Supplement with probiotics (friendly gut bacteria) powder or capsules added to food (1/8–1/2 teaspoon per day/up to 6 capsules) and digestive enzymes. Also add vegetable and fish oils. Pets with colitis may not be absorbing food completely and will need additional nutrients until they heal so add a good-quality, multi-mineral and vitamin supplement daily. One of the green super-foods, such as spirulina, and kelp add valuable nutrients (see Chapters 4 and 5).

Aromatherapy – Massage the intestinal area with a few drops of chamomile in a base oil.

Biochemical tissue salts – Use mag. phos. for cramping pains.

Herbs – Garlic helps to keep the right internal environment for the friendly gut flora and has an anti-spasmodic effect in the colon. Liquorice is also soothing and has an anti-inflammatory effect on the gut. Slippery elm is a wonderful long-term remedy for persistent problem and soothes and calms inflamed bowels and reduces flatulence. Fenugreek, peppermint, comfrey and aloe vera can also bring relief and ease discomfort.

Homoeopathy – Phosphorus.

Constipation

Constipation can be caused by a number of things, although incorrect diet is usually at the root of the problem. Not enough fibre in the diet is the commonest cause, but sometimes animals that have been eating bones get short-term problems and fur balls can cause constipation in cats (cats need regular grooming to avoid this problem). Lack of exercise and worm infestation are also considerations. If a change of diet does not sort the problem out then consult your vet, since more serious causes of constipation include cancer or a constricted bowel.

Symptoms of constipation in your pet include: straining to have a bowel movement, going for long periods between bowel movements (dogs and cats should go at least once or twice a day), hard, impacted faeces.

Long-term constipation can lead to more serious problems, such as bowel cancer, skin problems and obesity. If animals are not eliminating properly then they get a build up of toxic waste in the body which effectively poisons them and causes further health problems.

Diet – Change to a natural, preservative-free diet. Make sure they get a good balance of protein, whole grains and vegetables. Include lots of fibre in your pet's meal, such as brown rice, oats, raw grated vegetables (carrots, parsnips, beetroot, cabbage), prunes, figs (fresh or dried), grated apple. Oils, such as olive oil or sunflower oil (1/2–3 teaspoons daily), help to lubricate the bowel and alleviate constipation. Make sure your pet has access to fresh drinking water at all times. Supplement with probiotics daily, digestive enzymes and linseeds/flaxseeds (soaked overnight and added to food), a good-quality, multi-mineral and vitamin complex, plus additional vitamin C (500–5,000mg) which is a great cleanser.

Exercise – Sluggish animals can get constipated so make sure they get adequate exercise for their breed and age.

Aromatherapy – Massage the lower abdomen with olive oil and a few drops of sage, rosemary or marjoram.

Bach flower remedies – Use crab apple for cleansing. Stress, anxiety and emotional upsets can all cause constipation – refer to Chapter 11 for an appropriate remedy.

Biochemical tissue salts – Use nat. mur. for constipation alternating with diarrhoea.

Herbs – Aloe vera is cleansing and soothing, psyllium husks add fibre to the bowel and help to clear out toxic waste (1/2–2 teaspoons per day in food). If the constipation has been going on for a while, try one or more of the laxative herbs, such as rhubarb, senna pods or cascara sagrada.

Homoeopathy – Nux vomica is the basic constipation remedy. Give sulphur if there is also skin disorder, carbo. veg for simple constipation with gas and calc. carb. if the constipation is associated with eating bones and hard, chalky stools.

Diabetes

Diabetes is a disease of the pancreas that affects the body's ability to control its blood sugar levels. It is the pancreas's job to produce a hormone called insulin which keeps blood sugar levels balanced but, if this is not happening, glucose cannot be transferred from the blood for use in the cells. A diabetic animal will naturally drink more water to flush the excess sugar out of its system, but this also causes essential minerals and vitamins to be washed out, so although the animal may be eating plenty of food, it is also starving.

The main symptom of diabetes is excess thirst and frequent urination. Other signs and symptoms include lethargy, sugar in the urine and weight loss, despite a good appetite. Causes of diabetes include obesity, unhealthy diet (some commercial pet foods are high in sugar and preservatives), cortizone treatment, stress and shock.

Diabetes is a serious disease and should always be treated by a vet and your pet may need to have insulin injections for the rest of its life. Other health problems associated with diabetes include cataracts, liver and kidney disease, increased infections, heart disease.

Natural medicine and conventional medicine work well together to treat diabetes and there is much that can be done, especially with diet, to help control blood sugar levels and reduce or even remove the need for long-term use of insulin. Always let your vet know what you are doing, since insulin levels may need to be reduced in line with dietary changes. Never experiment with treating diabetes on your own without veterinary supervision.

Diet – A natural, preservative-free diet is essential along with additional supplements. The key word with diabetes is routine, so always make sure that your pet's meals are at the same time every day. Several small meals a day, rather than one big one, will also help with blood sugar control. Make sure the diet is based on whole grains (rice, millet, oats, corn meal), lean meats (chicken, turkey), eggs, fish, raw vegetables (carrots, green beans, alfalfa, Brussels sprouts, parsley, onions, garlic), plus supplements. Above all, avoid commercially prepared dog foods, especially the semi-moist ones as these contain high amounts of sugar and preservatives. The only way to be sure your pet's food is free of sugars and preservatives is to make it yourself from scratch (see Chapter 4).

Supplement the diet with digestive enzymes, a good-quality, multi-mineral and vitamin complex, brewer's yeast or a yeast free B complex and trace minerals, which are essential for blood sugar control, especially chromium (as glucose tolerance factor), zinc and manganese. Make sure these trace minerals are contained in your multi-mineral or add them according to body weight. Brewer's yeast contains manganese and chromium, and wheat germ contains chromium. Giving vitamin E (25iu–200iu daily) reduces the need for insulin. Also give vitamin C (500–5,000mg).

Exercise – Regular exercise is an important factor with diabetes. A diabetic pet needs a strict routine therefore try to exercise them at the same times every day.

Aromatherapy – Use eucalyptus and juniper, and lemon can be used for massage.

Bach Flower remedies – Hornbeam and olive can help to build up a weakened animal.

Herbs – Goldenseal helps to stabilise blood sugar levels and is the first choice of treatment. Garlic and liquid chlorophyll are also blood sugar balancers.

Homoeopathy – The main remedy for diabetes is syzygium.

Diarrhoea

Diarrhoea is not always a sign of illness. It has lots of causes, many of which are the body's natural way of getting rid of irritants such as food allergies, bacterial or viral infections, worms and toxins. In these cases, the diarrhoea usually stops once the toxins have been evacuated, and as long as there are no other signs of illness it is best to let nature take its course. Other factors, such as a change of diet or stress, can also bring on mild diarrhoea. Some animals will naturally seek out plants that will give them diarrhoea as a way of detoxifying their system. A short-term attack of diarrhoea is not usually a worrying sign, but continued diarrhoea is, and an animal can get very dehydrated and lose essential nutrients. If there is blood or mucus in the stools, tarry, black-coloured stools, or if the diarrhoea is accompanied by other symptoms of illness then take your pet to the vet. Puppies and kittens should always be taken to the vet at the first sign of diarrhoea since they can dehydrate very quickly and can even die without swift treatment.

Symptoms of diarrhoea are loose, watery stools and there may also be belching and wind. Sometimes blood and mucus, or undigested food is present in the stools and the animal may also vomit.

Mild, short-term diarrhoea can be treated at home, but long-term, serious problems should always be seen by your vet. If the diarrhoea continues for more than two or three days, a visit to the vet is essential.
Diet – At the onset of diarrhoea, the most important treatment is a day's fasting. Make sure your pet has plenty of water to drink though. Vegetable broths (the strained liquid only), brown rice water, barley water, apple-cider-vinegar water or honey water can all be given during the fast to support basic nutritional needs, while at the same time letting nature take its course. When giving food again, change to a natural preservative-free diet, since your pet may be sensitive to preservatives, colourings and others additives in commercially prepared foods. Plain boiled or steamed mashed potato helps to relieve diarrhoea and makes a good first meal following a fast day. Give probiotics and digestive enzymes daily, along with a good-quality, multi-vitamin and mineral complex once the fast has finished. If the diarrhoea persists then give activated charcoal tablets (see Chapter 16).
Aromatherapy – Chamomile, geranium and sandalwood can be added to olive oil and massaged into the abdomen to soothe the digestive tract.
Bach flower remedies – Use crab apple for cleansing.
Biochemical tissue salts – Use nat. mur. for thin, watery diarrhoea, or diarrhoea that alternates with constipation. Use nat. phos. for foul-smelling green stools, and combination S for stomach upsets.

Grapefruit-seed extract – Add 5–15 drops to food 3 times a day to help eliminate harmful bacteria or parasites. Start at a low dosage and gradually increase it until the diarrhoea has stopped.

Herbs – Garlic and goldenseal help to fight infections, slippery elm, as a syrup, powder or tea is soothing and nourishing, aloe vera juice is soothing and adds nutrients, parsley and fenugreek are digestive tonics. Meadowsweet is also an excellent herb for treating mild diarrhoea and marshmallow is soothing for intestinal inflammation.

Homoeopathy – Give arsen. alb. for watery stools, arsenic for vomiting and diarrhoea, merc. cor. for frequent diarrhoea with straining but no vomiting.

Flatulence

(Also see Stomach problems, Constipation, Diarrhoea in this section.)

Flatulence is caused by a build-up of gas in the stomach or intestines and can be accompanied by bloating, abdominal pain, belching and wind. Undigested food fermenting in the stomach is the commonest cause of excessive gas and it usually responds well to a natural preservative-free diet outlined in Chapter 4. In most cases a change of diet will be enough to sort out the problem. Food sensitivities can also cause flatulence. Give probiotics, digestive enzymes and stomach acid to assist optimum digestion. Activated charcoal granules/tablets also help relieve flatulence.

Aromatherapy – Peppermint can be massaged around the abdomen.

Biochemical tissue salts – Use mag. phos. or combination E for flatulence and indigestion.

Herbs – Aniseed, caraway, peppermint and fennel all help to reduce flatulence.

Homoeopathy – Use carbo. veg. for most cases, especially if foul-smelling, or nux vomica when accompanied by diarrhoea and digestive upset.

Foreign bodies

See First-aid use in Chapter 16.

Fur balls (cats)

Cats groom themselves much more often than dogs and are therefore more prone to swallowing their own hair, which gathers in the stomach forming hair balls. This is usually vomited up as knotted clumps of hair or passed out of their system in the faeces, especially if the cat's diet has adequate fibre and oils in it. The problem can become serious if their digestive system is weak or their nutrition inadequate, because then the hair balls can get stuck and act like a cork in their system – giving rise to diarrhoea followed by constipation, recurrent vomiting, lack of appetite, a build-up of toxins and, eventually, infection. You will know when your cat has a problem with hair balls when it vomits without bringing anything up, vomits foam without hair, or retches in an unsuccessful attempt to bring something up.

Prevention is always better than a cure. Regular grooming of cats, especially while they are moulting, reduces the amount of hair they might swallow.

Diet – Make sure their diet includes plenty of fibre, fats and oils to help the hair pass through the digestive system. Psyllium husks add fibre to the diet and help remove toxins from the bowel (see Chapters 4 and 5).

Herbs – Aloe vera juice helps to prevent constipation and has a healing and soothing action on the intestines.

Homoeopathy – Nux vomica is the primary remedy for hair balls and will help the animal to vomit or pass it through the bowel.

Liver disease

The liver has many and varied functions, including being a major player in the digestive process and in the elimination of toxins. Any liver condition, therefore, can have serious consequences and should always be seen by your vet first. However, there is a lot you can do with natural remedies that will support liver function and help it to regain health.

Signs of liver problems include vomiting, weight loss, odd-coloured stools, diarrhoea, increased thirst, swollen abdomen and lethargy.

Diet is the most important treatment for liver conditions, since a well-balanced natural diet can reduce the liver's digestive and detoxification workload. Chemical additives, artificial preservatives and colouring, medical drugs (eg worming tablets, flea powder), toxic metals and so on, all have to be processed by the liver; therefore the less of these your pet takes in, the better for its liver.

Diet – Change to a preservative-free, natural diet, avoiding red meats and milk. The diet should be made up of lean meats (include some organic liver), eggs, cooked whole grains, low in fats, and include raw vegetables (carrots and beetroot). Give a good-quality, multi-vitamin and mineral supplement daily, along with additional vitamin C (500–5,000mg daily), lecithin granules (1–3 teaspoons added to meals). Use only filtered or spring water, not tap water. Also add probiotics and digestive enzymes. Garlic, and apple cider vinegar are also helpful additions to the diet (see Chapters 4 and 5).

Aromatherapy – Rosemary and mint can be massaged around the liver area.

Bach flower remedies – Crab apple is cleansing. Use hornbeam for a sickly animal and impatiens for an irritable, touchy animal.

Herbs – Dandelion, burdock and milk thistle are gentle and supportive for the liver, milk thistle helps it to repair, swedish bitters are a liver tonic and can be found in health-food shops – mix it with some honey to make it palatable! Do not use herbal tinctures preserved in alcohol in cases of liver disease.

Homoeopathy – Use nux vomica for liver conditions and digestive upsets, chelidonium majus for jaundice and liver complaints.

Pancreatic problems

(See also Underweight and Diabetes in this section.) The pancreas has the job of keeping blood sugar levels stable. In terms of digestion the pancreas produces digestive enzymes that help to digest food. If it does not produce enough enzymes then you get a situation where your pet is literally 'starving in the midst of plenty' because it cannot digest and absorb nutrients properly. Symptoms include weight loss, diarrhoea, and lethargy. Many cases can be helped with a good-quality, natural diet and digestive enzyme supplements (see Chapters 4 and 5).

Stomach problems (gastritis)

(Also see Vomiting in this section.) Cats and dogs get upset stomachs just like us, and mostly it is not serious. The sort of things that cause upset are indigestion, eating food that has gone off (eg rubbish-bin raiding), swallowing hair, swallowing small hard objects, eating poisons (eg weedkiller), travel sickness and allergies. Other more serious causes can be liver, kidney or pancreatic disease or worms.

Gastritis is an inflammation of the stomach. Symptoms include being sick, along with one or more of the following: diarrhoea, abdominal pain, excessive gas, bloating, loss of appetite and listlessness. There may be fever in some cases.

Diet – The most important thing is to change your pet's diet to a fresh, preservative-free one. Food allergy is often the cause of stomach upsets, especially an allergy to cow's milk and wheat gluten. Your pet may have a weak intestinal system and be prone to upsets, in which case a natural, home-made diet will help to ease and strengthen their digestive system. Fasting for the first day or two of stomach upsets really helps to clear toxins out. (Follow the guidelines for fasting in Chapter 4.)

Once your pet is eating again digestive enzymes should be added to meals to aid digestion, plus a good-quality, mineral and vitamin supplement, brewer's yeast and probiotics (see Chapter 5).

Bach flower remedies – Use crab apple for cleansing, agrimony for indigestion caused by stress, hornbeam to help strengthen a sickly animal.

Biochemical tissue salts – Use combination S for stomach upsets.

Grapefruit-seed extract – Add 5–15 drops, 3 times a day to food to help eliminate harmful bacteria and parasites.

Herbs – Slippery elm is very soothing and healing and can be added to your pet's meals. Meadowsweet for stomach upsets. Chamomile and peppermint tea are also soothing for the stomach and help indigestion. Aloe vera helps to cleanse and soothe digestive problems. Parsley and dandelion are good digestive aids. Alfalfa, aloe vera and slippery elm offer extra nutrients as well.

Homoeopathy – Nux vomica is the classic remedy for digestive problems. Use arsen. alb. with accompanying diarrhoea, phosphorus where vomiting follows after eating, carbo. veg. for flatulence and foul smell.

Teeth and gums

Pets get tooth decay and gum disease just like us. However, the better their diet, the less likelihood there is of serious dental problems developing. If you give them sugary treats, then stop it now! Animals do not need them and are just as happy to munch on raw carrots or nutritious home-made biscuits (see Chapter 4).

It is a good idea to check your pet's teeth and mouth regularly for early signs of dental decay and gum disease. A build-up of tartar can lead to inflamed gums, infections and tooth decay. Some of the most obvious symptoms are bad breath, inflamed or swollen gums (gingivitis), bleeding gums, excessive salivation, loose teeth, build-up of tartar, pain when eating and loss of appetite.

Serious dental problems should always be treated by a vet, but there is a lot you can also do with natural remedies and a corrective diet at home. Prevention is the key word with dental problems.

Diet – Diet is the single most important factor in avoiding dental problems and keeping teeth and gums healthy. Raw food, which is hard and crunchy, added to their diet exercises teeth and jaws and helps to remove tartar. Raw, meaty bones are also essential for healthy teeth and gums. Cats that roam freely outside will naturally hunt for small animals and birds, eating the bones as well as the meat. Dogs and cats should be given raw bones regularly to chew on. For pets who cannot have bones, add bone-meal powder (1/8–1/2 teaspoon) to their food, adding extra calcium and phosphorus for healthy teeth. One of the best foods to give your pet regularly is raw meat, especially the tougher cuts like stewing steak or chuck steak, because it not only exercises the jaw but contains connective tissue which acts like dental floss! Raw meat can also help to scrape away some of the tartar (see Chapter 4). Dried food does not clean teeth and pets that are given a dried food diet often have the worst teeth.

A multi-mineral and vitamin supplement will build up the animal's general health. If there is a gum infection present, add additional vitamin C (500–3,000 mg daily) and raw garlic to their food.

Aromatherapy – Lavender and peppermint oils can be used externally for massaging inflamed or sore gums.

Biochemical tissue salts – Use calc. flour. to strengthen teeth.

Grapefruit-seed extract – Put a few of drops on a wet toothbrush to clean your pet's teeth as an effective infection fighter and preventative.

Herbs – Echinacea and Goldenseal tincture can be used directly on gums. They can also be taken in food to help boost the immune system and fight infection.

Homoeopathy – Use apis. mel. for swollen gums, hepar. sulph. for infected gums that bleed easily with a smelly breath, merc. sol. – a good all round remedy for gum disease.

Travel sickness

Most pets have no trouble travelling in the car or on a train but others can become anxious and fearful, and some are physically sick. Bach flower remedies will help with fears and anxieties related to travel, including air travel (see Behavioural problems in this chapter and also

Chapter 11) whilst there are a few natural remedies that can help with physical sickness. Also make sure your pet has access to fresh air while travelling.

Diet – A healthy diet generally will help to keep the digestive system in good condition. Do not feed your pet for at least an hour before travelling and make sure they have some fresh water available at all times.

Aromatherapy – A few drops of peppermint or melissa on your pet's blanket while travelling can help.

Bach flower remedies – Rescue remedy is the best all-round remedy for travel sickness combined with scleranthus. Air travel can be quite traumatic for pets, again rescue remedy will help. Also see Chapter 11 for remedies relating to specific fears or anxieties.

Biochemical tissue salts – Use kali. phos. for nervous sickness, nat. phos. for stomach upset.

Herbs – Ginger is the first choice for travel sickness. Fresh grated ginger can be added to home-made biscuits or given as tablets, capsules or tincture. Peppermint is also helpful and can be given as a tea or tincture half an hour before the journey.

Homoeopathy – Use cocculus given at least half an hour before travelling. Give ipecac for nausea and vomiting at least half an hour before travelling. Some of the homoeopathic suppliers make a travel sickness tablet for animals.

Vomiting

Occasional vomiting in cats and dogs is quite normal since they get upset stomachs just like us, but frequent or repeated vomiting is a sign of a more serious problem. Occasional vomiting can be caused by a number of things including fur balls, stomach upsets, and food or plant material getting stuck in the throat. Sometimes animals intentionally eat grass to make themselves sick as a way of cleansing their system.

More serious cases of vomiting, which might bring up blood, can indicate an infection, worms, liver, kidney or pancreatic disease, poisoning or digestive problems and should always be checked out by your vet.

Diet – The best treatment for a sick animal is to fast them for 24 hours to let their system clear of toxins. You can leave a bowl of vegetable broth or rice water available for them to drink, as well as fresh drinking water (see fasting in Chapter 4). An animal that has been sick will often be dehydrated, so they need to have plenty of fluids. Once they begin to eat again, the first few meals should be bland and easy to digest. Add a good-quality, multi-mineral and vitamin supplement to their food for a few weeks. Vomiting can rob the body of important nutrients and these need to be replaced. Add probiotics to rebalance the internal environment. Activated charcoal helps to soak up toxins.

Aromatherapy – Lavender or peppermint can be massaged into the abdomen or used in a diffuser/burner.

Bach flower remedies – Crab apple is the cleansing remedy. Use olive for physical exhaustion. Hornbeam for fatigue and to help build up a sickly animal.

Biochemical tissue salts – Use ferr. phos. for vomiting undigested food, nat. sulph. for bile, combination S for stomach upsets.

Grapefruit-seed extract – Give 5–15 drops in food, 2 or 3 times daily.

Herbs – Slippery elm powder in food helps to soothe the stomach. Aloe vera juice is soothing and healing and provides nutrients. Chopped mint leaves are soothing and can be added to their food or given as a tea.

Homoeopathy – Use nux vomica for occasional vomiting associated with stomach upset. Use phosphorus if they are sick immediately after food, arsen. alb. for vomiting with diarrhoea.

Weight problems
This includes loss of weight, overweight, obesity.

Overweight/obesity
Animals in the wild are rarely overweight, but it is a common problem with domestic pets. Between 25–30% of dogs are overweight; some are obese. Cats are less prone to becoming overweight; none the less, fat cats do exist! Overfeeding, allergies, constipation and incorrect diet are usually at the root of the problem, therefore diet is the most important thing to be looked at. There are other causes of weight gain, including heart disease, liver disease, kidney disease and an underactive thyroid. Therefore it is best to get a vet's diagnosis first to eliminate more serious causes. Overweight animals are less healthy and more prone to illness than thinner animals, and obesity puts excessive strain on the heart and other organs and can lead to problems such as arthritis, rheumatism, diabetes, and lowered immunity. Obese animals have a much shorter life expectancy as well.

Diet – Changing to a natural preservative-free or allergy diet is essential, and this may be enough on its own to return your pet to its optimum weight without reducing its food intake. Many commercial pet foods are high in sugars and fat and provide less than nutritious calories which may cause your pet to overeat. Avoid giving lots of titbits and treats between meals and don't feed your pet from the table – this sets up bad habits which are hard for everyone to break! An overweight animal is often overloaded with toxins and has a sluggish eliminative system, so a day's fast on a weekly basis can really help in the first few months of treatment (see Chapter 4 for dietary guidelines).

Give a good-quality, multi-mineral and vitamin supplement. Kelp tablets assist the metabolism and have a cleansing action on the body. Add psyllium husks, digestive enzymes and probiotics for a sluggish digestive system (see Chapter 5).

Exercise – Make sure your pet is getting regular exercise appropriate to its breed and age.

Herbs – Seaweed stimulates the metabolism and can be helpful with weight loss or an underactive thyroid. You can buy dried seaweed which can be cooked in with a brown rice diet or use kelp tablets/powder. Aloe vera juice is a rich source of nutrients and intestinal cleanser and helps relieve constipation. Dandelion and parsley to help get rid of water retention. Milk thistle will help to assist a sluggish liver.

Underweight

Weight loss can be caused by a number of things including allergies, worms, inadequate digestion (malabsorption), incorrect diet, overactive thyroid, not enough food, cancer, liver disease, pancreatic disease, infections, emotional upsets such as loss or grief or following a major trauma like an operation. With cats, there is always the finicky eater syndrome to consider, and this may just take time and patience to introduce them to a new and healthier way of eating. As a first step, it is always best to get a vet to check your pet for any serious underlying problems, especially if the weight loss happens suddenly.

Diet – Diet is the key to weight gain once any serious underlying problems have been addressed. Change your pet's diet to a natural preservative-free diet including plenty of raw food. The following foods can be added to their meal to encourage weight gain: oats (porridge), olive oil, sunflower oil or corn oil, goat's milk, goat's or ewe's milk yoghurt, brewer's yeast, wheat germ, dried fruit, eggs. Cats can have butter added to their food as well. Watercress helps to promote digestion. Initially you may have to give your pets several small meals a day while you are building them up. Also give digestive enzymes, probiotics and a good-quality, multi-mineral and vitamin supplement, royal jelly capsules. In cases of inadequate digestion, alfalfa and apple cider vinegar assist the absorption of nutrients (see Chapter 5).

Bach flower remedies – If your pet has gone off its food because it is grieving or stressed, then flower remedies can help to rebalance their emotional state. Read Chapter 11 and choose one or more of the remedies that suit your pet's emotional state. Use beech for picky, finicky eaters, especially cats.

Herbs – Try using fenugreek seeds (1/2–3 teaspoons). These can be boiled up with brown rice or soaked in hot water overnight and the seeds and liquid added to food. Fenugreek smells of curry and your pet will too, but most cats and dogs love the taste! It is a good digestive tonic. Mint also aids digestion.

EAR PROBLEMS

Ear problems are common in both cats and dogs and include ear mites (see Parasites), discharge, wax, smelly ears, irritation, inflammation, and infections.

Signs and symptoms of ear problems include frequent head shaking, scratching, clawing or pawing at the ears, rubbing the ears on the ground, discharge, heat, inflammation, irritation – and sometimes the ears can smell like sweaty socks or a ripe cheese!

Ear problems can be caused by a number of things, including grass seeds getting caught in the ear, allergies, injuries, infections (fungal, bacteria, or yeast). Many of the flop-eared type dogs, like spaniels and setters, are prone to ear infections because their ears are closed from the air, becoming a perfect environment for fungus and bacteria to multiply. If something gets stuck in the ear accidentally then get your vet to remove it, since poking around in an animal's ear can damage it.

Ear problems can be cleared up very effectively using natural remedies, and the sooner the problem is caught the better. Left untreated, ear infections can spread to other areas of the body.

Suitable treatments include acupuncture, aromatherapy, diet and food supplements, healing, herbs and homoeopathy. Before treating your pet at home read the relevant chapters for information on treatment, remedies, dosage, suppliers etc.

Diet – A preservative-free natural diet will enhance your pet's health and help to clear up infections and boost the immune system. Ear problems caused by allergies should also clear up once your pet is changed to an allergy-free diet. Vitamins A and E, and zinc help to heal skin problems. Follow the diet and supplement recommendations in Chapters 4 and 5. Diluted grapefruit-seed extract, apple cider vinegar or lemon juice in water can be used to clean out the ears of flop-eared dogs and help to fight against bacteria and infections. Check their ears regularly for grass seeds and infections and to give their ears some fresh air, pin them back occasionally with a clothes peg.

Aromatherapy – Tea tree oil and garlic oil have anti-fungal and anti-bacterial properties and can be used with olive oil/sweet almond oil to clean out infected ears. Add a couple of drops of tea tree oil to two or three ounces of olive/almond oil and put this in the affected ear. Massage gently for a few minutes and then wipe the ear to remove any excess oil. This also helps to bring wax and sticky discharges to the surface and can dislodge foreign bodies that have got stuck. Almond oil and olive oil soften and dissolve dark waxy discharges and are soothing and healing. You can also add some vitamin E to the oil mixture which is also soothing and healing.

Bach flower remedies – Use crab apple for cleansing and detoxifying, hawthorn for run-down animals.

Grapefruit-seed extract – Mix 12 drops with an eggcup of oil to clean out the ears (see Aromatherapy above). This is highly effective against yeasts, fungal and bacterial infections.

Herbs – Aloe vera juice can also be used for cleaning and fighting infections and has a soothing effect on painful ears. Put two or three ounces of liquid into the affected ear, massage for a few minutes and then clean out any excess with cotton wool. Witch hazel is soothing and can be used to clean infected or inflamed ears. Goldenseal fights infection and boosts immunity. You can use goldenseal tincture to clean out infected ears. Calendula lotion can be used to soothe irritated or inflamed ears.

Homoeopathy – Use hepar. sulph. for inflamed ears, sensitive to touch, graphites for smelly discharges, rhus tox. for chronic ear infections, hepar. sulph. for offensive smelly discharges, merc. sol. for suppurating ears with smelly discharge, silicea for recurrent ear infections. Calendula tincture can be diluted in warm water with sea salt to clean the ears.

EYE PROBLEMS

Eye problems in cats and dogs should always be seen by a vet first so that you know what the trouble is. Depending on what is wrong, there is much that can be done for the eyes using natural therapies and remedies. Common eye problems include cataracts, conjunctivitis, injuries, failing eyesight. Suitable treatments for eye problems include acupuncture, aromatherapy, diet and food supplements, flower essences, healing, herbs, homoeopathy.

Before treating your pet at home, read the relevant chapters for information on treatment, remedies, dosage, suppliers etc.

Cataracts

Cataracts are fairly common in older pets and are recognisable as a cloudy white or blue film over the eye which can eventually lead to blindness. They can be caused by injury, allergies, diabetes and infections but many health professionals feel they are a result of internal toxins and malnutrition. Diet is a vital part of the healing process and a pet brought up on a natural diet will probably never have cataracts. In many cases, changing to a natural preservative-free diet will arrest the progress of cataracts.

Diet – Follow the guidelines for a natural preservative-free diet and supplement programme in Chapters 4 and 5 including vitamins A, C and E. Zinc is an essential mineral for eye health. Raw cucumber can be used over the eye or the juice used for bathing.

Herbs – Eyebright can be made into a tea and the strained and cooled liquid used as an eye wash. It can also be taken internally, added to food. Aloe vera juice is a good internal cleanser and can also be used diluted in water as an eye wash for around the eye.

Homoeopathy – Silica delays the progress of mature cataracts, cineraria tincture diluted can be used as an eye drop. Calc. carb. for old, overweight pets.

Conjunctivitis

Conjunctivitis is an inflammation of the tissue around the eye and is common in both cats and dogs. The usual causes are something getting into the eye, allergy, infection, or an irritant. Dogs that stick their heads out of car windows on journeys can get conjunctivitis if something flies into their eye. Signs of conjunctivitis are red, sore-looking eyes with a runny discharge.

Diet – Change to a natural preservative-free diet and supplement programme outlined in Chapters 4 and 5 to keep your pet healthy and strong. Zinc is a good supplement for healing eye problems. Slices of cucumber held over the eye can cool hot, inflamed eyes, or the juice can be used as eye drops.

Aromatherapy – Soak some cotton wool in tepid water with a few drops of chamomile added and hold over the eye.

Herbs – Tea made from eyebright or goldenseal can be used to bathe around the eye. Vitamin E can be added to the liquid to enhance the healing process. A pad of cotton wool soaked in witch hazel can be held over shut eyes. Eyebright and goldenseal can be taken internally as well.

Homoeopathy – Use euphrasia eye drops diluted in water for bathing the eye. Use euphrasia (tablets) for profuse watering or infected eyes, apis. mel. for sudden attacks and swelling, argent nit. for uncomplicated cases.

Injuries

Eye injuries are pretty common, resulting from fights, accidents, foreign bodies getting into the eye and bruising.

Diet – A good, healthy diet and supplement programme will help with the healing process (see Chapters 4 and 5). Slices of cucumber can be held over the eye, or use the juice as an eye drop.

Herbs – Eyebright and goldenseal can be used externally as a tea to clean round the eye. They can also be taken internally. Cotton wool soaked in witch hazel used externally is soothing, held over a shut eye.

Homoeopathy – Arnica ointment can be used around the eye externally to reduce swelling or taken internally as tablets. Calendula lotion gently rubbed around the eye can soothe and relieve pain. Use euphrasia eye drops diluted in water for bathing the eye. Eye drops (natural if possible) bought from your local pharmacist are also very effective in reducing inflammation and preventing infection.

Failing eyesight

Old age is often accompanied by failing eyesight and many older pets develop cataracts (see above). There is little you can do to prevent naturally degenerating eyesight; however the Bach flower remedies can help your pet adapt to change and cope with progressive loss of sight, especially if they become nervous or fearful with it (see Chapter 11).

IMMUNE SYSTEM AND INFECTIOUS DISEASES

An animal's immune system protects it from infectious diseases like kennel cough and distemper. A healthy immune system will be able to defend the animal against viral, bacterial or fungal invasions, whereas a weakened immune system will not. This is a key point in understanding why some animals become infected and others do not, since infectious agents are always around, but only those with weakened defence systems become ill. As Louis Pasteur said on his death bed, *'seed is nothing, soil is everything'*.

Many of the infectious diseases that affect cats and dogs can be fatal; therefore it is vital to take your pet to the vet if you suspect an infection. Some of the more common infectious diseases include parvo virus, distemper, kennel cough, lyme disease, canine hepatitis, feline leukaemia virus, feline infectious peritonitis, feline immunodeficiency virus, chlamydia (cats), ringworm, skin diseases, wound infections. Immune system diseases include autoimmune problems, such as allergies, asthma, skin complaints and cancer.

Many things can weaken the immune system and leave a pet vulnerable to disease, including stress, chemicals and food additives, toxic metal poisoning, air pollution, poor diet, frequent or multiple vaccinations, chemical flea powders and unhealthy lifestyle. Our pets are frequently getting diseases that were rare 30 years ago, and many people would put this down to an increased stress on the immune system. Prevention is the best protection, therefore it is a good idea to give your pet immune-boosting remedies at times of stress, such as before and after being vaccinated, if they are unwell, before and after an operation, or if they are under emotional stress. Pets that are fed a natural preservative-free diet and regular supplements are far less likely to become infected, and more likely to recover if they do become ill.

Signs that your pet has an infectious illness are runny, watery eyes, coughing, sneezing, loss of appetite, listlessness, vomiting, diarrhoea, and a fever. The earlier the infection is caught the easier it is to cure.

Natural treatments and remedies are highly effective in boosting and strengthening the immune system and maintaining resistance to infectious diseases. However, always take your pet to see the vet since infectious diseases can be fatal. Let them know what natural treatment approach you wish to follow and get a referral. Suitable treatments include acupuncture, aromatherapy, diet and food supplements, flower essences, healing, herbs, homoeopathy.

Before treating your pet at home read the relevant chapters for information on treatment and remedies, dosage, and suppliers etc.

Diet – A natural preservative-free diet and supplements are the cornerstone of a healthy immune system, whereas a bad diet invites disease (see Chapter 4 for details). Fasting is really helpful when there is a fever or at the onset of an infection. Garlic is the number one infection-fighter and immune-system supporter, so add up to three raw cloves daily to food. Also add probiotics, digestive enzymes and a green super-food. If you only add one supplement, make it vitamin C. It helps to rebuild the immune system and is a good preventative measure against infections. Use high quantities of vitamin C spread throughout the day (you can go to bowel-tolerance levels). Other immune-boosting supplements are the B vitamins, A and D (or use cod liver oil), zinc, magnesium, calcium, vitamin E and selenium. Apple cider vinegar added to food or water is also an immune booster, as is royal jelly. Do not use brewer's yeast in cases of fungal or bacterial infections. Acorn Supplements Ltd (UK) make a wonderful veterinary supplement called Immune Plus which combines immune-boosting vitamins, minerals, trace elements and herbs (see Chapter 5).

Aromatherapy – Immune-boosting oils include lemon, sage, eucalyptus, thyme, tea tree and bergamot. They can be used diluted for massage or in a burner or diffuser. Eucalyptus burned daily in a kennels or cattery situation can help prevent the spread of diseases, such as kennel cough.

Bach flower remedies – Use rescue remedy at the onset of symptoms, crab apple for cleansing, hornbeam to strengthen, olive for very ill, weak animals. There are many other potent flower essences from around the world that are helpful in fighting infections (see Further reading, Chapter 11).

Grapefruit-seed extract – Add 5–15 drops to food 3 times a day. Grapefruit-seed extract is a potent antibiotic and anti-microbal. Its natural antibiotic action helps to boost the immune system.

Herbs – Give cat's claw, echinacea or astragalus to boost the immune system. Garlic has powerful anti-viral, anti-bacterial and anti-fungal properties and can be given in large quantities (up to 3 raw cloves a day). St. John's wort also has reputed anti-viral properties. Aloe vera is a liver cleanser and digestive aid. Other liver-supportive herbs include milk thistle, dandelion, parsley and red beet powder. Nutritious herbs include alfalfa, oat straw, horsetail and ginseng.

Homoeopathy – Use aconite at the start of symptoms, belladonna for fevers, gelsemium for flu-like symptoms, distemper.

KIDNEY AND URINARY PROBLEMS

The kidneys, bladder and urinary tract make up the urinary system, which can be prone to bacterial infections and degenerative disease. It is crucial that the urinary system stays healthy, since it is responsible for removing waste products from the body, particularly the by-products of protein metabolism. Protein in the urine is a sure sign that there is something wrong with the kidneys. Some of the more common problems affecting cats and dogs are cystitis, bladder and kidney stones, kidney disease and incontinence. Suitable treatments include acupuncture, aromatherapy, biochemical tissue salts, diet and food supplements, flower essences, healing, herbs, homoeopathy.

Before treating your pet at home read the relevant chapters for information on the treatment, remedies, dosage, suppliers etc.

Bladder/kidney stones and gravel

Bladder and kidney stones are formed out of mineral salts and can cause intense discomfort to an animal. Inadequate diet and lack of fluids are the most common causes, therefore a good-quality natural diet is a simple preventative measure. Stones and gravel tend to form more often in the bladder than in the kidneys and cause recognisable symptoms like recurrent cystitis, incontinence and difficulty urinating. There may be blood in the urine.

Much can be done with natural treatments and remedies to prevent stones from developing, especially with a foundation of a natural diet and supplement programme.

Diet – Change your pet's food to a natural preservative-free diet. Make sure they also have plenty of fresh water available, preferably filtered or bottled water. Dried food should never be given to pets with bladder or kidney stones since it is thought to be a major contributing factor. The

▼

phosphorus content of the diet should be kept low which means giving your pet high-quality protein (chicken and turkey, occasionally, red meat) and fish. Dogs can also have eggs, yoghurt, tofu and beans. Avoid poor-quality protein such as meat by-products and meat derivatives found in most commercially prepared pet foods. Add apple cider vinegar to their food or water to acidify the urine. An acid urine can dissolve gravel and small stones. Other positive foods include brown rice, potatoes, asparagus, cranberries and cranberry juice (unsweetened only),carrots and oat flakes.

High quantities of vitamin C help to acidify the urine and dissolve stones. Vitamin C also detoxifies the body and reduces the likelihood of stones forming. Also add vitamin E, cod-liver oil (or vitamins A and D), magnesium, calcium and vitamin-B complex (see Chapters 4 and 5).

Aromatherapy – Use juniper, sandalwood and ylang ylang.

Bach flower remedies – Use crab apple for cleansing.

Biochemical tissue salts – Use mag. phos. and calc. phos. given together.

Grapefruit-seed extract – Use 3–12 drops, 2 or 3 times a day, added to food. This is a very potent remedy.

Herbs – Use couchgrass, uva ursi and sarsparilla. Parsley, nettle and dandelion are also helpful herbs.

Homoeopathy – Use calc. carb. for overweight heavy animals, calc. phos. for lean animals.

Cystitis

(See also Immune system and infectious diseases in this chapter, Bladder/kidney stones, above.) Cystitis is an uncomfortable and painful infection of the urinary tract and tends to be more common in cats than in dogs. It has noticeable symptoms including an urgent need to urinate, frequent urination but not passing much; there can be a fever, and sometimes there is blood in the urine. Cystitis is often recurrent and if unchecked can lead to more serious kidney infections. It is usually caused by a bacterial infection or bladder stones. Natural treatments and dietary changes can greatly help alleviate the problem and prevent recurrence.

Diet – Follow a natural preservative-free diet and supplement regime outlined in Chapters 4 and 5. Don't feed dried foods to pets with cystitis. Cystitis is rare in animals that are fed a natural home-made diet. In acute cases, a day of fasting on barley water and parsley water cleanses the system and fights bacteria. Try to encourage your pet to drink plenty of water. Cranberry is a very effective treatment for cystitis and can be given as juice (unsweetened only), in capsules or in powder form. Unsweetened cranberry juice acidifies the urine and makes it inhospitable for bacteria to thrive. Probitotics and high levels of vitamin C (given throughout the day) are also recommended.

Aromatherapy – Use juniper, tea tree, sandalwood and bergamot.

Bach flower remedies – Rescue remedy.

Biochemical tissue salts – Use kali. mur., kali. phos., mag. phos.

Grapefruit-seed extract – 5–15 drops added to food 2 or 3 times a day as a powerful anti-microbal and anti-biotic.

Herbs – Use horsetail, uva ursi and nutrient herbs, such as dandelion, parsley, watercress and nettles.

Homoeopathy – Use cantharis for acute cystitis, given as soon as the first symptoms appear.

Feline urology syndrome (FUS)
The symptoms are similar to cystitis (including depression, loss of appetite, straining to pass urine) and should be checked out by your vet. It is caused by tiny crystals blocking the flow of urine from the bladder which can lead to cystitis and even kidney failure. Never feed dried foods to a cat with FUS. These are prone to dehydrate an animal's system and also the protein quality in dried foods is low, which causes the urine to be alkaline. An alkaline urine encourages the growth of unfriendly bacteria and the formation of stones and gravel. (Also see Cystitis and Bladder/kidney stones in this section.)

Incontinence
It is a very upsetting experience for pets to be incontinent as they don't like upsetting their owners by urinating in the home or missing the litter tray. Unless the animal is quite elderly, incontinence is usually a symptom of bladder or kidney infection, and these should be checked out first. Incontinence can sometimes have an emotional problem at its root (see Behavioural problems). It can also be caused by spaying, and repeated infections like cystitis. (See also Cystitis in this section and Immune system and infectious diseases in this chapter.)

Diet – Follow the guidelines for a natural preservative-free diet with no dry foods, milk, or yeast. Include plenty of raw vegetables in their food, eg carrots, green beans, asparagus. Apple cider vinegar adds potassium. Barley water assists urinary function (also see Bladder/kidney stones in this section). Add the B vitamins, vitamin C, cod-liver oil (or vitamins A and D), vitamin E, zinc, calcium, magnesium and probiotics to their diet. Unsweetened cranberry juice or cranberry capsules assist the urinary system, and is especially effective when combined with vitamin C and probiotics (see Chapters 4 and 5).

Aromatherapy – Use juniper.

Bach flower remedies – Use hornbeam for strengthening.

Herbs – Use parsley, nettles, dandelions, horsetail.

Homoeopathy – Causticum for weak bladder muscles, calc. flour. for young animals, apis mel. for pets that can't make it outside or to the litter, sulphur for incontinence and frequency.

Kidney disease

The main function of the kidneys is to eliminate waste, maintain the body's fluid balance and control blood pressure. Kidney problems are fairly common in older cats and dogs, particularly kidney failure which is slow and progressive.

Signs and symptoms of kidney disease are gradual weight loss, lethargy, lack of appetite, bad breath, increased thirst, poor coat condition, smelly coat, inability to hold urine overnight and vomiting. Repeated bouts of cystitis can eventually lead to kidney disease, which is one of the leading causes of death in cats. Skin problems are often associated with kidney disease and can later precede kidney failure.

Always take your pet to the vet if you suspect kidney disease, as it can be serious if not treated. Natural medicine has a lot to offer, especially in the area of nutrition.

Diet – Natural treatment involves helping the kidneys to do their job therefore the less toxins that are in your pet's diet the less strain there will be on the kidneys. Change to a natural preservative-free diet and supplement regime. Cut out all salt. The protein content of their diet should be low but make sure it is good quality protein ie. not meat by-products, meat derivatives, etc. Do not use dried food, as this can lead to dehydration and the low protein quality of dried food can lead to cystitis, FUS, and kidney and bladder stones.

Fresh filtered or bottled water should be available at all times. Barley water is a good kidney cleanser. Other helpful foods for the kidneys are potatoes, green beans, celery, asparagus, parsnips (raw, grated) and green leaf vegetables. Supplement the diet with B complex, vitamin C, cod-liver oil (or vitamins A and D), calcium and magnesium. Apple cider vinegar added to water or food adds potassium. Also give small amounts of linseed/flaxseed oil. A good-quality, multi-mineral and vitamin supplement (see Chapters 4 and 5).

Aromatherapy – Use juniper and bergamot.

Bach flower remedies – Use olive for weak, exhausted animals, crab apple for cleansing.

Biochemical tissue salts – Nat. mur. helps with fluid balance.

Herbs – Nettles and parsley are gentle diuretics and help the kidneys remove waste. Couch grass, horsetail and uva ursi are helpful for the kidneys. Alfalfa adds a wide range of nutrients.

Homoeopathy – Use nux vomica to reduce toxicity, phosphorus for acute kidney disease with vomiting, nat. mur. for increased thirst and poor skin condition.

MUSCLE AND JOINT PROBLEMS

Muscle and joint problems include arthritis, rheumatism, hip dysplasia, bone fractures, sprains and strains, dislocation, slipped disc, spinal problems and paralysis. Suitable treatments include acupuncture, aromatherapy, biochemical tissue salts, chiropractic, diet and supplements, flower essences, healing, herbs, homoeopathy and T-touch.

Before treating your pet at home, read the relevant chapters for information on treatment, remedies, dosage, suppliers etc.

Arthritis (osteoarthritis and rheumatism)

Arthritis is an inflammation of the joints, mostly affecting older pets, and can be crippling and extremely painful. The two most usual forms of the disease are osteoarthritis and rheumatism. Dogs tend to be affected more than cats.

Signs and symptoms of arthritis in your pet include stiffness, especially after rest, aggravated symptoms in cold, damp weather, difficulty jumping up or climbing stairs, lagging behind on walks, soreness hours after exercise, swollen or painful joints and lameness.

Nutrition is the key element in the holistic prevention and treatment of arthritis to the extent that animals brought up on a natural preservative-free diet seldom suffer from this disease. Arthritis is often a result of frequent or multiple vaccination, poor nutrition with hereditary factors.

Arthritis is a whole-body disease and therefore needs an holistic approach to treatment. Because it is an autoimmune disease, emphasis is on boosting the immune system and improving the overall health of the animal as well as encouraging elimination of toxins. Toxins settle in the joints, making the problem worse, therefore detoxification needs to be part of treatment. Holistic treatment may not bring about a complete cure, but it can slow its progression and give your pet a much more comfortable life. Arthritis is a chronic disease, therefore natural therapies require patience and commitment since treatment will be long-term.

Structural therapies like chiropractic are of great help in all musculo-skeletal problems. Acupuncture and healing also help greatly with pain relief, boosting the immune system and stimulating self-healing. If you do decide to opt for the natural approach remember that steroid drugs should only be phased out under veterinary guidance.

Diet – Change to a natural preservative-free diet that includes plenty of raw vegetables, easily digested protein eg fish, eggs, chicken, turkey, plus (for dogs) live yoghurt, cottage cheese and tofu, cooked whole grains eg brown rice, and pure fresh water, not tap water. Potatoes, tomatoes and peppers can aggravate arthritis, so avoid feeding these. Fasting for one day a week helps to remove toxins from the system. During the fast you can give your pet carrot and celery juice, barley water, rice water or vegetable-broth water. If your pet is overweight this puts extra strain on joints and ligaments and speeds up degeneration (see Weight problems, in this chapter).

Glucosamine sulphate helps bone cartilage to rebuild, leading to greater joint mobility and pain relief (give 250–1,000mg, 3 times daily for up to 3 months, then reduce the dose to twice a day). Also add cod-liver oil (1/2–3 teaspoons) daily for 6 months. Acorn supplements Ltd (UK) make an excellent veterinary supplement called Osteo Ease which I have had consistently successful results with. It includes herbs, vitamins, minerals, amino acids and biochemicals to help relieve pain, improve mobility, repair damaged tissue and strengthen the immune system. Other helpful additions to the diet include apple cider vinegar (1/2–3 teaspoons), a yeast free vitamin-B complex (1–3 tablets), kelp (1–3 tablets), vitamin C (500–7,000mg), vitamin E (50–300iu), bone-meal, wheat-germ oil (1/2–2 teaspoons) lecithin (1/2–2 teaspoons), green-lipped mussel and a good-quality, multi-mineral and vitamin complex. Add one of the green super-foods, plus kelp to cleanse and nurture the system. Older pets or those with digestive problems may also need digestive enzymes. As a preventative measure, it is really important to give good nutrition to pregnant females (to protect their young from developing arthritis by providing a natural diet and additional vitamin C). See Chapter 5 for food supplements and Chapter 17 for pregnancy and associated problems.

Exercise – Moderate, regular exercise related to your pet's breed, and plenty of sunshine and warmth. Dogs benefit from swimming in the sea but make sure they are dried well afterwards so that they do not sit around damp and cold.

Aromatherapy – Massaging the affected areas using essential oils is soothing to stiff and painful joints and increases the circulation. Beneficial oils include juniper, eucalyptus, birch, thyme, rosemary and pine. Add a few drops of one or more essential oils to a base of olive oil or sweet almond oil.

Bach flower remedies – Use crab apple for cleansing and detoxifying, hornbeam for strengthening.

Biochemical tissue salts – Use calc. flour., nat. phos. and nat. sulph. Use silica for inherited joint pains, combination M for rheumatic pain.

Herbs – The following herbs help to reduce inflammation and relieve pain – garlic, feverfew, devil's claw, cleavers and ginger. Alfalfa, aloe vera and chlorophyll help to cleanse toxins from the body. Use cat's claw to boost the immune system. Liquorice root is a natural anti-inflammatory. Other herbs that can be added to food include the green leaf herbs, such as nettles, dandelions, watercress and parsley, which are all good detoxifiers. (Parsley, and watercress are also high in vitamin C.) Comfrey is the bone-healing herb. One herb that seems to stand out on its own in the treatment of arthritis is boswellia, which is highly anti-inflammatory and anti-pain. A combination of slippery elm and cayenne in a 10:1 ratio can be mixed into a paste with water and used as a poultice.

Homoeopathy – Rhus tox. is the 'classic' arthritis remedy for stiffness on getting up, that eases with movement, but is worse in cold, damp weather. Give bryonia when pain is worse for movement, arnica for swelling or bruising, calc. carb. for old, stiff, overweight pets.

Broken bones and fractures

Broken bones and fractures are usually caused by accidents, particularly being hit by a car, but they can also be caused by brittle bone disease (osteoporosis). Osteoporosis is a thinning of the bones usually caused by inadequate diet or kidney disease. As the bones become more brittle it leaves the animal susceptible to fractures and breaks.

The signs and symptoms will be pretty obvious especially if the fracture has penetrated the skin. Other signs include misshapen bones and joints, swelling and lameness.

Fractures and breaks need immediate veterinary attention. If you have the Bach flower rescue remedy or homoeopathic aconite to hand then give one or both of these to reduce the shock and trauma. Once the bones have been reset, natural remedies and treatments can speed up the healing process and support recovery.

Acupuncture and chiropractic are particularly helpful in treating broken bones and fractures.

Diet – A good-quality diet and supplements regime will help to heal bones and speed recovery. Give plenty of vitamin C (double dose), bone-meal, glucosamine sulphate (250–1,000mg 3 times daily for 3 to 4 months, then reduce to once or twice a day).

Bach flower remedies – Give rescue remedy for shock and trauma.

Biochemical tissue salts – Calc. flour. and calc. phos. given together.

Herbs – Comfrey is known as the 'bone-knitting' herb and can be taken internally or used externally as a poultice. It also helps to reduce bruising. Comfrey ointment can also be applied externally. Hilton Herbs (UK) do a ready-made comfrey compress. Alfalfa, horsetail grass and oat straw add calcium to the diet for bone healing. A poultice of fresh mullein leaves can also be used.

Homoeopathy – Give aconite immediately for shock and trauma, followed by arnica for bruising. Symphytum (comfrey) promotes healing and knitting of bones. Silicea strengthens the skeleton. Give calc. carb. for heavy, overweight animals, calc. phos. for thinner animals.

Hip dysplasia (dogs)

Hip dysplasia is a malformation of the hip's ball-and-socket joint. It affects one or both hips and can lead to a complete loss of use of the hind legs. It is particularly prevalent among large breeds like German shepherds, labradors and retrievers. As the dog gets older it also becomes more prone to getting arthritis and rheumatism in the affected legs.

Symptoms of hip dysplasia are stiffness, a wobbly gait while walking, sitting down a lot, and generally being out of sorts. Although the causes are thought to be hereditary, many holistic vets feel that generations of inadequate diet (particularly a lack of vitamin C) is the main cause of hereditary hip dysplasia. Natural treatments can help to prevent the problem recurring in future generations and ease the condition for dogs that are already suffering. Acupuncture, healing and chiropractic are all good treatments for hip dysplasia along with dietary changes and a good supplement programme.

Diet – Change to a natural preservative-free diet as outlined in Chapter 4. Pregnant bitches and puppies need additional vitamin C (500–5,000mg for adults, 50–100mg for puppies under six months old) and raw, meaty bones or bone-meal daily. Acorn Supplements Ltd (UK) make an excellent veterinary supplement called Osteo Ease (also see dietary recommendations for arthritis).

Bach flower remedies – See Arthritis.

Essential oils – See Arthritis.

Herbs – Use comfrey and white willow bark for pain relief (dogs only), aloe vera.

Homoeopathy – Give conium for advanced hip dysplasia, calc. carb. for fat, young dogs, calc. phos. for lean, thin dogs.

Joint dislocation

The most usual causes of dislocated joints are road traffic accidents or falls. Veterinary treatment is essential, but you can also give your pet the Bach rescue remedy or homoeopathic aconite as a first-aid measure to reduce shock and trauma.

Signs and symptoms of dislocated joints are usually easy to see, such as misshapen joints, lameness and stiffness around the joint.

Once the joint has been put back into place, natural remedies and treatments will help speed recovery. A pet with damaged joints is more prone to getting arthritis at a later date. Acupuncture, healing and chiro-practic are particularly good treatments. (Also see Hip dysplasia and Arthritis.)

Diet – A good-quality, natural diet and supplement programme are vital for speedy recovery. Give vitamin C (double dose) to heal damaged tissues, glucosamine sulfate (250–1,000mg, 3 times daily) for cartilage and joint repair and maintenance of healthy joints, raw, meaty bones or bone-meal for added calcium.

Bach flower remedies – Give rescue remedy as a first-aid measure for shock and trauma.

Biochemical tissue salts – Use calc. flour. and calc. phos. together.

Herbs – Comfrey, horsetail grass, oat straw and kelp will all help with joint-healing and recovery.

Homoeopathy – Give aconite as a first-aid measure for shock and trauma, arnica for bruising, hypericum for pain relief.

Paralysis and spinal disease (spondylosis, spondylitis, slipped disc)

Spinal diseases and accidents involving the spine often lead to paralysis. Spinal diseases include spondylosis, spondylitis and slipped disc and are more common in dogs than in cats. They tend to be degenerative, becoming more apparent with age.

Breeds of dog with long bodies and short legs, such as basset-hounds and dachshunds, are particularly prone to spinal problems, as are some larger breeds like German shepherd dogs. In cats, spinal problems are usually related to accidents.

Spondylitis is a degenerative disease of the spine that causes pain and inflammation and is essentially arthritis of the vertebrae (see also Arthritis). As it progresses, there is increased bone formation and the joints fuse together causing curvature of the spine. This becomes a chronic condition known as spondylosis.

Slipped disc is caused by the degeneration of a disc which then presses on the spinal cord, causing severe weakness and paralysis.

Some of the causes of spinal problems, other than accidents, are inadequate diet, lack of exercise and stress. Therefore much can be done as a preventative measure. Signs and symptoms include rigidity of the spine and pain on getting up, progressive paralysis of the back legs, loss of strength at the rear end, muscle wasting, curvature of the spine, loss of control of the bladder or bowels.

Acupuncture, chiropractic and healing are highly recommended.

Diet – A good-quality diet and supplement programme are essential for keeping the musculo-skeletal system healthy (see Arthritis and Chapters 4 and 5 for details). Vitamin C (high dose) strengthens connective tissue, cartilage and bone. Also give vitamin E (300–600iu) and use castor oil as a compress for pain and swelling.

Exercise – Light exercise is important if the animal can manage. Swimming is a wonderful way to exercise the body.

Aromatherapy – Lightly massage with the following oils: lavender, marjoram and rosemary.

Biochemical tissue salts – Give silica.

Bach flower remedies – Use hornbeam and olive to strengthen weak animals, rescue remedy and star of Bethlehem for injury.

Herbs – Use scullcap, valerian and feverfew for pain relief and as a relaxant. Use white willow (dogs only) or liquorice for inflammation, alfalfa, horsetail grass and oat straw to strengthen bones and joints, comfrey and scullcap to repair nerves and relieve pain.

Homoeopathy – Give nux vomica for slipped disc, pains, spasms and paralysis, arnica for swelling or bruising, ruta grav. for slipped discs or injuries affecting the vertebrae, conium maculatum for rear-end paralysis.

Sprains and strains

Most active pets are likely at some time to suffer from sprains or strains, such as pulled or torn muscles, overworked muscles, stretched ligaments or swollen tendons. Signs of this in your pet include limping, holding up a paw, localised swelling, and signs of pain.

Diet – A good-quality diet and supplement regime help to promote healing and speed recovery. Additional vitamin C helps to heal tissue and reduce inflammation. Calcium and magnesium help to reduce muscle spasms and pain. Osteo Ease (Acorn Supplements Ltd) given for a few weeks will help relieve inflammation and pain. Fasting for 24 hours on just honey water also promotes healing (see Chapters 4 and 5).

Aromatherapy – Massaging the affected area with one or more of the following oils diluted in a base oil will ease pain and reduce inflammation and stiffness: birch, lavender, eucalyptus, juniper, rosemary.

Bach flower remedies – Give rescue remedy for shock.

Biochemical tissue salts – Use ferr. phos. or combination I for rheumatic pain.

Herbs – Comfrey can be taken internally or used as a cold compress. Hilton Herbs (UK) make a wonderful veterinary comfrey compress. Alfalfa, horsetail and oatstraw add calcium for strains. Witch hazel can be used as a compress to reduce swelling and bruising. Herbal creams can be used externally, such as arnica for bruising, ruta for injury to ligaments, and rhus. tox. for injury to muscles with swelling and stiffness. Tiger balm used externally also soothes sprains and strains.

Homoeopathy – Give arnica for bruising and pain, pulled tendons and ligaments with stiffness and pain. A cold compress of diluted arnica tincture is helpful in reducing swelling. Use rhus. tox. for persistent lameness, sore, stiff, swollen muscles, ruta grav. for injury, pulled muscles, sprains and strains.

OPERATIONS

There may come a time when your pet needs to have an operation; however there is a lot you can do both before and after to help the healing process and avoid infection. The emphasis is on boosting the immune system so that your pet's powers of recovery are strong. If the operation isn't sudden, begin to support your pet's immune system for at least two weeks beforehand. (See also Immune system and infectious diseases, Spaying and neutering, in this chapter, and Wounds in Chapter 16.)

Diet – A natural preservative-free diet is the foundation of a strong immune system. Your pet will have to fast for a short period before the operation and it's a good idea to fast them for 12–24 hours afterwards as well. This gives the body a rest from digesting food so that it can put its resources into recovery (see fasting guidelines in Chapter 4). Garlic is the number one infection-fighter and immune-system supporter – add up to three raw cloves daily. Always add probiotics if your pet has had a course of antibiotics. Other important supplements include digestive enzymes, green super-foods, vitamins A, C and E, zinc and fish and vegetable oils. A good-quality, multi-nutrient formula like The Missing Link, Pet Plus will contain most of the above. Acorn Supplements (UK) make an excellent supplement called Immune Plus, which combines immune-boosting vitamins, minerals, trace elements and herbs (see Chapter 5).

Aromatherapy – Immune-boosting oils include lemon, tea tree and bergamot. These can be diluted in a base oil and used for massage, or used in a burner or diffuser near your pet's bed. Ylang ylang and rosemary are revitalising. Tea tree is cleansing and antiseptic and can be used diluted to clean the wound.

Bach flower remedies – Rescue remedy will help to calm an animal before and after the operation. Clematis helps them to recover after an anaesthetic, hornbeam for strengthening.

Grapefruit-seed extract – This is a potent natural antibiotic and can be used to clean the operation wound and prevent infection. Use 12 drops diluted in an eggcup of boiled and cooled water, twice a day. Grapefruit-seed extract capsules can be taken internally as well, as a natural antibiotic.

Herbs – Astragalus, cat's claw and echinacea are all good immune-boosting herbs. Give up to three raw cloves of garlic daily as well. Milk thistle supports the liver and detoxifies the body after an anaesthetic. Aloe vera also has great cleansing properties and is a good digestive aid.

Homoeopathy – Give arnica before and after the operation to reduce bruising, hypericum helps to relieve pain and repair damaged tissue. Hypericum and calendula tinctures can be used diluted with water to clean the operation wound.

PARASITES

Parasites are creatures that live in or on your pet, such as worms and fleas. They are unwelcome lodgers, since they take as much as they can and give nothing back in return. Most pets at some time will be host to a parasitic invasion; however, healthy cats and dogs with a strong immune system will naturally eliminate them and are unlikely to be bothered by parasites for long. A natural, preservatve-free diet and a healthy lifestyle are two of the most important front-line defences against these unwelcome guests.

Some of the most common parasites that affect dogs and cats are fleas, ticks, lice, mites and various kinds of worms. Although there are plenty of chemically prepared flea powders and flea collars on the market, these contain toxic elements and repeated use can harm your pet. Many commercial flea treatments can aggravate asthma and be a contributing factor in certain types of cancer and nervous disorders. Many worming preparations can be as toxic to your pet as they are to worms! However, there is a lot you can do at home to prevent parasites in the first place, and natural treatments and remedies can help to eliminate the problem. Suitable treatments include acupuncture, aromatherapy, biochemical tissue salts, diet and supplements, flower essences, healing, herbs and homoeopathy. Before treating your pet at home, read the relevant chapters for information on treatment, remedies, dosage, suppliers etc.

Ear mites

Ear mites live in a cat's or dog's ear canal and cause inflammation, irritation and a thick, brownish-red crust. They are common in cats and dogs and often spread from one to the other. Signs to look out for are lots of head shaking, along with excessive scratching and rubbing of their ears. Use a torch and check their ears for a dry crumbly brown discharge inside the ear canal. See fleas for general advice on treatment at home.

Specific treatment – Olive oil with a few drops of grapefruit-seed extract and vitamin E added can be poured into the ear and massaged for a while to loosen any crusty material and bring it to the surface. After a few minutes clean out the ear with cotton wool. You can also clean the ear with garlic water (fresh garlic boiled in water, strained and cooled), diluted tea tree oil or apple cider vinegar. Never stick anything hard inside the ear in an attempt to clean it or delve deep into the ear canal. Clean the ears every day for at least a week. If the ears are very red and inflamed, calendula cream will help to sooth them. Also clean around the ears with a herbal shampoo and use a herbal flea powder (see Chapter 13 for details).

Bach flower remedies – Crab apple will help to expel impurities.

Homoeopathy – Use sulphur for hot, red, smelly ears.

If the mites persist then consult your vet.

Fleas

Although fleas can affect any pet, the healthier it is the less likely it is to become infested. Fleas prefer animals in poor health with lowered immune systems and are usually only a nuisance in warm weather. During the summer months check your pet regularly for fleas. Apart from being able to see them, other signs to look out for are scratching, chewing and biting, licking their coat and pulling out hair. Some animals may have an allergic reaction to flea bites or have red and sore skin. Sometimes you can see flea dirt, which is dry, black and dust-like, on light-coloured animals.

Tapeworms are carried by fleas, so if your pet is infested with fleas they may also have worms.

Diet – A natural preservative-free diet will improve your pet's general health and enhance its immune system. Raw garlic is one of the best anti-parasite treatments – chop it up and put it in your pet's food or use garlic tablets/capsules if they don't like the taste, 1 clove for cats and small dogs, 2 cloves for medium dogs and 3 cloves for large dogs. Brewer's yeast is also an excellent repellent. This can be mixed into their food (1 teaspoon daily for cats and small dogs, 2 teaspoons for medium dogs, and 3 teaspoons for large dogs). Both garlic and brewer's yeast should be given for at least 4 weeks. Brewer's yeast can also be rubbed into your pet's coat and used as a natural flea powder. Add zinc (5–20mg daily) to help boost the immune system, vitamin C (500–5,000mg daily) to detoxify and boost the immune system. Use a yeast-free B-complex supplement if your pet is allergic to brewer's yeast (see Chapters 4 and 5). Also see Immune system, in this chapter.

Environment – If you find fleas on your cat or dog you can be sure that ten times that amount are hiding in its environment! Eggs and larvae need to be eliminated as well, therefore flea control means cleaning and vacuuming all the places your pet sleeps and lies. Regular cleaning and grooming interrupts the flea's life cycle and makes breeding more difficult.

Aromatherapy – Lavender, lemon and peppermint deter fleas and you can spray a mixture of these essential oils mixed with vodka and water on your pet's bed or fur as a deterrent. Other useful oils include eucalyptus, cedar, cypress and lemon. These can be massaged into their coat in a base oil and then combed through with a flea comb. You can also put a few drops of essential oil on your pet's collar for a home-made natural flea collar.

Bach flower remedies – Use crab apple for cleansing.

Grapefruit-seed extract – Add 10–20 drops to a cup of water and massage or comb through your pet's fur. It can also be used in a spray bottle to spray your pet's bedding.

Herbs – Mint leaves, lavender seeds, rosemary and sage can be left in and around your pet's bed to deter fleas. Cat's claw or echinacea taken internally will help to boost the immune system. Garlic given regularly also helps to expel parasites. You can buy herbal flea powders or make up your own by mixing together powdered herbs like wormwood, eucalyptus, mint, rosemary, sage and yellow dock. Ask your herbalist to make up a powder for you. This can be rubbed into their fur and combed through every day for about four weeks or until all the fleas have gone. (Remember to do this outside so that escaping fleas remain outside!) Garlic powder can also be rubbed into their fur. Acorn Supplements Ltd (UK) make an excellent herbal flea powder called Flea Clear, plus a veterinary supplement to be taken internally if the infestation is stubborn to clear (see Chapter 5 under Useful information).

Homoeopathy – Use pulex for flea allergies and flea infestation, sulphur where the skin is dry and flaky, scratching.

Grooming – Regular grooming is essential where external parasites are concerned. Get a special flea comb from the pet shop and thoroughly groom your pet from head to toe. (Again, remember to do this outside so that any fleas that drop off are left outside!) Essential oils and herbal flea powders can be combed into the fur at the same time.

Bathing – Fleas hate a clean coat therefore bathing helps to prevent infestation and gets rid of existing fleas. There are several natural pet shampoos on the market or you could use garlic and lemon water. (Garlic and lemon water are easily made by boiling crushed cloves of fresh garlic and a whole lemon in water and using the cooled liquid.) Make sure you wash really well around the head and ears which is where fleas tend to like. Keeping your pet clean and well-groomed is essential when dealing with external parasites.

Lice

Lice are tiny insects that can be seen on the animal's fur – as can their eggs. A pet with lice will be restless and rub and scratch its skin. Follow the treatment recommendations for fleas.

Mange

This is caused by tiny mites that burrow into the animal's skin. It is mostly found in dogs, but can affect cats too. Mange is a sign that the animal's immune system is under par. These parasites are difficult to remove and need veterinary guidance; however, follow the advice given for fleas to help boost your animal's general health, speed up their recovery and prevent recurrence. Also see Immune system, in this chapter.

Ticks

Ticks are temporary parasites that burrow into the skin of warm-blooded animals to feast on their blood. They vary in size, from a few millimetres in length to a centimetre long when fully swollen with blood. Only the head end burrows into the skin and the body can be easily seen on the surface. Once they have eaten they usually fall off the host. However, tick bites can get infected, so it is best to remove ticks as soon as you notice them on your pet. (If they do get infected follow the treatment advice for abscesses.) See Fleas for general treatment.

Removing a tick – Heat the end of a blunt knife in boiling water and press it onto the tick's body, being careful not to burn your pet's skin. The tick can then easily be pulled out with some tweezers. It is important to kill the tick before trying to get it out otherwise its head can get left in and cause an infection. A dog breeder friend of mine says she has great success removing ticks using a dab of gin. Leave it on for a few minutes then carefully pull the tick out using tweezers.

Aromatherapy – Dab the tick with eucalyptus oil or camphor and then wait about a minute before pulling the tick out. Always make sure the whole tick is removed. Tea tree oil can be dabbed on the wound to prevent infection and to help the skin to heal.

Grapefruit-seed extract – Put a few drops of grapefruit-seed extract directly onto the tick. Remove the tick and put another drop on the bite to prevent infection.

Worms

Various types of worms can affect dogs and cats, but the two most common are roundworm and tapeworm. They both live in the intestinal tract and can be seen in the faeces. Roundworms look like coiled springs and can also be seen in an animal's vomit, especially with young animals. Tapeworms are flat and segmented and the segments look like grains of white rice in the faeces or around the anus. A flea-infested animal should also be checked for tapeworms.

Pets most at risk from worms are newborn kittens and puppies (they can be passed from the mother), pets infested with fleas, animals that eat wild creatures and pets that are old or run down.

Apart from seeing worms in the faeces, other signs that your pet has worms are weight loss, excessive appetite or lack of appetite, bad breath, bloated abdomen, bony body, vomiting, irritation around the anus, diarrhoea and a general decline in health.

Conventional worming treatments are chemical-based and can be harmful in the long run. Try natural treatments first and use preventative measures on a regular basis. Continual worming with conventional products can weaken your pet's immune system.

Diet – Diet is one of the most important factors in treating worms. The healthier your pet is the more resistant it will be to a parasitic infestation. Change to a natural preservative-free diet. One of the most potent treatments is raw garlic added daily to food (1/2–2 cloves depending on the animal's size). Other beneficial foods that can be added to meals include pumpkin seeds (1/4–2 teaspoons), dried coconut (1/2–2 teaspoons), grated carrots (1/2–2 tablespoons) and dried figs (1–3 figs chopped). Oat bran or psyllium husk powder (1/2–2 teaspoons) are an important addition as roughage helps to carry worms out of the intestines. Fasting your pet for a day at the beginning of treatment is also helpful. As a regular preventive treatment, use raw garlic, oat bran or psyllium husks, raw carrots, beetroot or turnips, pumpkin seeds or sesame seeds, wheat-germ oil (1/4–1 teaspoon) and dried figs.

Pets with worms will be deficient in nutrients, so get them onto a good multi-mineral and vitamin formula. Make sure this contains zinc, iron, vitamin-B complex, vitamin A and vitamin C. Vitamin C is a great detoxifier and can be given in addition to a multi-nutrient formula (500–5,000mg daily) (see Chapters 4 and 5).

Bach flower remedies – Use crab apple for cleansing, hawthorn for vitality.

Grapefruit-seed extract – This is a highly effective treatment for worms and can be given on a reglar basis as a preventative measure. Give 5–15 drops, 2 or 3 times daily in food for 6 weeks.

Herbs – Use large amounts of garlic (up to 3 raw cloves a day), aloe vera, parsley, wormwood, black walnut hull and cloves.

Dr Hulda Clark's herbal parasite cure for pets:

1. Parsley water: Cook a big bunch of fresh parsley in 4 pints of water for 3 minutes. Throw away the parsley. Freeze most of the parsley water in small containers for later use. Put 1/2–2 teaspoons parsley water on your pet's food daily, for a week.
2. Black walnut hull tincture: Use 1 week later, putting 1 drop on the food. Treat cats only twice a week; treat dogs daily (1–3 drops).
3. Wormwood capsules: 1 week after the black walnut tincture start the wormwood. Open the capsule and put a tiny pinch on their food every day or a bigger pinch for large dogs.

4. Cloves: Begin this 1 week after the wormwood. Put a tiny pinch on their food, or a bigger pinch for large dogs.

By the fourth week your pet will be having parsley water, black walnut hull tincture, wormwood and cloves daily. Keep this up for another 3 to 4 weeks. If they get reinfested then repeat the regime from the beginning. The parasite cure can be given to your pet annually as a preventative measure.

This parasite cure for pets is taken from *The Cure For All Diseases* by Hulda Regehr Clark, PhD, ND; ProMotion Publishing.

Homoeopathy – For roundworms use cina or chenopodium. For tapeworms use granatum, felix mas. Arbrotanum can also be given.

PREGNANCY AND ASSOCIATED PROBLEMS

Pregnancy is a time of high nutritional need when the animal not only needs more food but also a good, well-balanced supplement regime. If the female is in peak health there is a much better chance that all the offspring will be healthy and the pregnancy and labour problem-free. Nutrition is the most important factor in keeping your pet healthy throughout the pregnancy. Natural treatments and remedies can help to alleviate problems that do arise, such as false pregnancy, inadequate milk production, infertility and mastitis.

There are plenty of good books detailing the ins and outs of breeding; this section is only aimed at listing the remedies and treatments that can positively assist pregnancy. Please read other books for detailed advice on breeding.

Suitable treatments include acupuncture, aromatherapy, biochemical tissue salts, chiropractic, diet and supplements, healing, herbs, homoeopathy and T-touch. Before treating your pet at home, always read the relevant chapters for information on treatment, remedies, dosage, suppliers etc.

Many of the commonly used essential oils and herbs should not be used during pregnancy, so always be sure which ones are safe to use when treating your pet at home.

Abortion

See Pregnancy, in this section.

False pregnancy

With a false pregnancy, a bitch can have all the symptoms of a real pregnancy without actually being pregnant. The signs are easily recognisable, including greater hunger, swelling of the abdomen, milk production, restlessness – and she may go as far as making a nest for herself. Some dogs take things into their nest to look after and can be quite aggressive if you try to take away their 'phantom pups'. The most common cause of a false pregnancy is hormonal imbalance. Sometimes this can be triggered by emotional factors (see also Chapter 11 and Behavioural problems earlier in this chapter).

Diet – A good-quality diet and supplement programme help to bring the body back into balance. Soya milk or tofu can be added to the diet, along with evening primrose oil and vitamin E to help balance the hormones (see Chapters 4 and 5).

Bach flower remedies – Use holly for aggression, mustard for mood swings, walnut to help them adapt to change.

Herbs – Agnus castus helps to balance the female hormones. Add 5–20 drops of tincture to food, 2 or 3 times a day.

Homoeopathy – Use sepia for aggressive or moody females, pulsatilla for symptoms that vary.

Inadequate milk production

Sometimes the female is not producing enough milk, or there may be no milk flow at all, which leaves a litter of hungry pups waiting to be fed. This can be caused by a hormonal imbalance, stress or mastitis (also see Mastitis). Natural treatments and remedies can help to stimulate milk production and bring the body back into balance.

Diet – Chicken, oats and artichokes (artichoke hearts can be bought in tins or jars) have milk-stimulating properties and can make up a large proportion of the animal's meal. For general advice of nutrition and supplements follow the recommendations given for pregnancy (also see Chapters 4 and 5).

Herbs – Fennel, milk thistle and fenugreek seeds stimulate milk production.

Homoeopathy – Pulsatilla can be given during labour to help stimulate milk production or after labour if there is inadequate milk.

Infertility

Infertility can be caused by a number of factors, including poor diet, nutrient deficiencies, hormonal imbalance, stress, heavy toxic load, obesity, problems with the reproductive organs and, of course, unsuccessful mating or infertility in the stud dog or tom-cat.

A good-quality diet and supplement programme are fundamental and can be enough on their own to turn round infertility, since nutrient deficiencies are a common cause. Structural causes may also be a part of the problem, therefore you might want to consider chiropractic as well.

Things to avoid prior to pregnancy are X-rays, steroid drugs, vaccines, and antibiotics.

Diet – Change to a preservative-free natural diet, using as many organically grown ingredients as possible and fresh bottled or filtered water, not tap water (see Chapter 4).

Add a higher dose than usual of supplements including vitamins A, C, D, and B complex (or brewer's yeast). Vitamin E is especially important when treating infertility. Also add zinc, magnesium, calcium, fish oil and evening primrose oil (see Chapter 5).

Bach flower remedies – Use clematis for animals lacking in energy, hawthorn to strengthen.

Herbs – Use agnus castus to help balance the female hormones. Raspberry leaf helps to strengthen the womb and reproductive system. Add alfalfa, or another of the green super-foods, and kelp for their rich nutrient content.

Homoeopathy – Use sepia for unpredictable, aggressive animals, pulsatilla for quiet, shy animals.

Mastitis

Mastitis (swollen mammary glands) is caused by a bacterial infection and animals are most susceptible to it when they are producing milk. The infected breast will be hard, sensitive and often red or purple in colour. Other symptoms to look out for are abscesses, fever, loss of appetite and depression. (Also see the Immune system.)

Diet – Follow the guidelines for a natural preservative-free diet and supplement programme outlined in Chapters 4 and 5.

Aromatherapy – Chamomile, geranium, peppermint and rose can be used to make an oil and water compress and held on the affected areas.

Bach flower remedies – Use hornbeam for strengthening, crab apple for cleansing, mustard for depression.

Grapefruit-seed extract – Add 5–15 drops of grapefruit-seed extract to your pet's food daily to kill harmful bacteria. Diluted grapefruit-seed extract can also be used externally as a wash, 3 times daily.

Herbs – Comfrey, slippery elm and poke root can be used as a soothing poultice. Use echinacea to help fight infection, poke root for infections and to reduce inflammation, cleavers for swollen glands. Peppermint can be used as a cold compress on hot, swollen teats.

Homoeopathy – Use aconite for the first signs of mastitis, belladonna when there is also fever and redness, bryonia for hot, painful and hard breasts worse for touch or movement. Phytolacca is an all-purpose mastitis remedy.

Pregnancy

Pregnancy is a time of great nutritional need and cats and dogs will need more food and a good supplement regime throughout. Good nutrition is the key to a successful pregnancy and trouble-free delivery. It helps to prevent birth defects, runt litters, and complications during and after labour. Before deciding to breed from your female, make sure she is fit and well. Pre-pregnancy health is of the utmost importance for both the males and females to ensure a litter of strong and healthy offspring.

Diet – Diet is the most important thing to be considered. We know, for example, that vitamin C helps to protect against hip dysplasia in dogs, and garlic can prevents worms in newborn kittens and pups. During pregnancy huge nutritional demands are made on the female as new animals are being formed and continual breeding without attention to diet and supplements can leave an animal depleted and nutrient-deficient. As the pregnancy progresses, give her several small meals throughout the day rather than one big one. Follow the dietary recommendations in Chapter 4 and give a little more food than usual. (Nursing mother's will also need more food than usual.) Avoid chemicals, preservatives and drugs, such as commercial fleas powders and worming tablets. Fresh bottled or filtered water should be available at all times.

Give a good-quality, multi-vitamin and mineral complex – again give her a higher dose than usual. Make sure the supplement includes vitamins A, B complex, C, D and E. Wheat-germ oil is a good source of vitamin E, and cod-liver oil provides vitamins A and D. You may have to add extra vitamin C on top of the multi-vitamin (1000mg–7,000mg of vitamin C daily). Calcium, magnesium and zinc are also important minerals. Add vegetable oil (or butter for cats) and cod-liver oil. The protein quantity can be slightly increased for both cats and dogs, making sure it is good-quality protein including eggs, goat's milk, liver, cottage cheese, yoghurt, meat and fish. Oats are good for exhaustion after labour and help to strengthen the body. Kelp, the green super-foods and watercress are good sources of vitamins and minerals and can be added to the diet. The pregnant female may also need some digestive enzymes added to food to help with digestion as the pregnancy progresses (see Chapter 5 for supplements).

Aromatherapy – It is best to avoid essential oils during pregnancy. Post-labour, clary sage and jasmine help to ease the pain of the birth.

Bach flower remedies – Give rescue remedy during and after labour, oak for exhaustion. Clematis helps newborn puppies and kittens to wake up and breathe. Use walnut to help the mother adjust, crab apple for cleansing after the birth.

Herbs – Raspberry leaf is traditionally used during pregnancy and helps to make labour and delivery easier. Use nettles to strengthen and support the whole body (good source of iron and vitamin C). Post labour, use comfrey and horsetail for healing, milk thistle, fenugreek and fennel to help the flow of milk if there is poor milk production. (Herbs to avoid during pregnancy include aloe vera, wormwood, juniper, sage and strong laxative herbs.)

Homoeopathy – Caulophyllum given 3 to 4 weeks before the birth can ease labour (1 tablet daily). Using pulsatilla during labour promotes milk production, eases the birth and calms the mother. Use aconite for fear or shock, arnica for bruising and overexhaustion.

RESPIRATORY SYSTEM

Respiratory problems range from a stuffy nose and a cough to cat flu and bronchitis. Although cats are more prone to these sorts of problems than dogs, when a lot of dogs are kept in a confined space, such as boarding kennels or dog shows, they can catch an infectious cough called kennel cough. There are many causes of respiratory diseases (infections, allergies, asthma, heart disease, parasites) – some of which, such as kennel cough, are serious – so always get your pet checked out by a vet so that you know exactly what is wrong. Most minor respiratory diseases respond well to natural remedies and there is much you can do to relieve your pet's condition. Suitable treatments include acupuncture, aromatherapy, diet and supplements, flower essences, healing, herbs and homoeopathy. Before treating your pet at home always read the relevant chapters for information about the treatment, the remedies, dosage, supplies etc. The following are a few of the more common conditions which will benefit from natural remedies:

Cat flu

See Immune system and infectious diseases.

Coughs

There are many types of cough and many underlying causes. Some coughs are dry (no mucus) and others wet (involving bringing up mucus). Coughing is the commonest symptom of respiratory problems and can be brought on by a range of things including infections (viral, bacterial, fungal), allergies, irritants, heart disease, lung congestion and parasites. Many pets also suffer from the adverse effects of their owner's smoking. The most common type of cough in dogs is kennel cough, which is an infectious viral disease. The dog may not appear to be ill, other than having a harsh, dry cough which is persistent and irritating. Cats can have a similar harsh, dry type of cough which may indicate bronchitis. Less serious coughs may be a result of a cold and repeated infections indicate that their immune system needs a boost.

Diet – Fasting is one of the most beneficial treatments for dogs or cats with an infectious cough or any virus-based respiratory disease, such as kennel cough and cat flu (also see Immune system and infectious diseases). Raw garlic is a wonderful anti-viral and can be added to a pet's food, or given in capsule form when fasting. Change your pet's diet to a natural preservative-free diet. Supplement the diet with vitamin A (5–10,000iu daily) to heal mucus membranes, vitamin C (500mg–5,000mg daily), vitamin E (50–100iu daily) and zinc (5–20mg daily) to boost the immune system. Cod-liver oil given on a daily basis is also helpful (see Chapters 4 and 5).

Aromatherapy – Eucalyptus is the main oil for respiratory diseases. In this case it is best used in a diffuser/burner placed near your pet twice a day for about 15 minutes. In kennels or catteries, burning eucalyptus oil daily is a great preventative measure against infections. Other useful oils include, tea tree, pine and myrrh.

Bach flower remedies – Use crab apple to cleanse, hornbeam to strengthen, olive to give physical strength to an exhausted animal.

Biochemical tissue salts – Use ferr. phos. for acute, dry coughs, kali. sulph. if worse in the evening, mag. phos. if it is worse for lying down or convulsive bouts of coughing, combination J for all coughs.

Grapefruit-seed extract – Add 5–15 drops to food, 3 times a day. Grapefruit-seed extract and Echinacea tincture combined make a great cure for coughs.

Herbs – Use garlic, liquorice, coltsfoot, golden seal, cat's claw, echinacea, sage, thyme. Garlic is a good all-round infection fighter. Goldenseal fights infection and cat's claw is a good immunebooster. You can also buy ready-made herbal cough mixtures from herbalists and health-food shops. These usually contain herbs like liquorice, comfrey, coltsfoot, slippery elm and mullein and can be given in the following dosage: cats and small dogs – infant's dose, medium dogs – child's dose, large dogs – adults dose. You can mix cough mixture with some raw honey to make it more tasty for your pet.

Homoeopathy – Use arsen. alb. for harsh coughing that worsens at night, bryonia for dry coughing that worsens with movement, aconite at the onset of coughing to stop it progressing further.

Kennel cough
See Immune system and infectious diseases, and Coughs.

Stuffy nose, runny nose, sinusitis, sneezing, colds, catarrh
Colds and nasal problems are usually caused by infections (bacterial or fungal), allergies (cigarette smoke, dust, house-dust mites) and sometimes tumours. Apart from obvious symptoms like sneezing and mucus discharges, your dog or cat may shake their head a lot too and be generally out of sorts. Cats are more prone to catarrhal problems than dogs.

Diet – Feed a natural diet free of preservatives. Garlic helps to destroy mucus and can be added raw to your pet's food. Raw, grated beetroot and carrots help to cleanse the body. Ginger helps to eliminate mucus from the sinuses. Supplement the diet with vitamin C (500–5,000mg daily), vitamin A (10,000iu daily), vitamin E (10–100iu daily) and zinc

(5–20mg daily) (see Chapters 4 and 5).

Aromatherapy – Use eucalyptus, olbas oil, tea tree, thyme. These are best used in a diffuser/burner and placed near your pet twice a day for at least 15 minutes at a time. This will help to clear the nasal cavities.

Bach flower remedies – Use olive for an exhausted, run-down animal, hornbeam for strengthening, crab apple for cleansing.

Biochemical tissue salts – Combination Q for catarrhal sinus disorders, nat. mur. for watery clear discharges, calc. flour. for thick, yellow discharges, combination J for flu-like symptoms.

Herbs – Use goldenseal, garlic, liquorice, comfrey, fenugreek.

Homoeopathy – Use gelsemium for sneezing, runny nose, fever and raw throat. Kali. bich. is a good remedy for catarrhal symptoms, pulsatilla for conjunctivitis with catarrhal symptoms.

SKIN AND COAT

Skin and coat problems are very common amongst dogs and cats and seem to be on the increase. The skin is the largest organ in the body and one of the routes through which toxins are eliminated. Skin problems often indicate toxic overload, allergies, immune-system compromise, frequent or multiple vaccinations, parasitic or bacteria infection. If the process of elimination through the skin is suppressed with steroids and antibiotics the toxins are likely to be driven deeper, causing more serious problems at a later date. Diet is one of the most important factors in skin diseases and poor coat conditions and should be the first thing that is looked at. Much can be done just by correcting your pet's diet to a more natural one. In some cases, a day's fast on a weekly basis can help, since it gives the animal's system a rest and promotes the elimination of toxins. Skin complaints can sometimes be difficult to shift completely, but you can go a long way towards keeping things under control using natural remedies and dietary changes.

The following are some of the more common skin and coat problems that your pet may encounter, many of which can be treated at home. If your pet is suffering or the condition is too serious for home treatment, consult your vet.

Suitable treatments include acupuncture, aromatherapy, biochemical tissue salts, diet and supplements, flower essences, healing, herbs and homoeopathy.

Before treating your pet at home it is important to read the relevant chapters on the treatments and remedies you are choosing to use and for information on dosage and suppliers etc.

Abscesses

An abscess is a small amount of pus trapped under the surface of the skin. Usually they form after a bite or wound heals over, trapping bacteria or dirt inside which then becomes infected. You will notice signs of infection by a red, swollen area of the skin that feels hot to the touch. It may also be painful. If the abscess is in your dog's or cat's mouth, they may also be off their food and generally out of sorts. (Mouth abscesses should be checked out by a vet in case dental treatment is needed.)

In order to heal, an abscess needs to be burst so that the puss can escape, bringing the infected material with it, and then the wound should be thoroughly cleaned. To draw out the puss, use hot compresses 3 or 4 times a day for 15 minutes at a time using warm, salty water with a few drops of tea tree oil added. Use 1 teaspoon of sea salt to a cup of warm water. A friend of mine swears by a bread poultice to draw out pus.

Diet – A natural preservative-free diet will help enhance the animal's immune system and self-healing ability. A good-quality, multi-mineral and vitamin supplement for cats or dogs should be taken daily plus additional zinc and vitamin C to help with the healing process (see Chapters 4 and 5).

Aromatherapy – Tea tree and thyme can be dabbed on the affected area. Lavender and tea tree can be used as a warm compress on the abscess. Raw honey can also be spread on the abscess to draw out the pus.

Biochemical tissue salts – Use silica for an abscess ready to burst or that has already burst.

Grapefruit-seed extract – A powerful anti-bacterial and antibiotic used externally as a wash. Add 10 drops to an eggcup of oil or water and apply twice a day to the affected area.

Herbs – Garlic, cat's claw and echinacea boost the immune system and will help with the healing process. Comfrey is also an important infection-healing herb and can be used externally as a compress or taken internally. Liquid garlic can be used to clean around the abscess. This can be bought ready-made or make your own by liquidising a clove of garlic in a cup of water. A paste of slippery elm powder will help to draw out the pus.

Homoeopathy – Use hepar. sulph. if the abscess is actively discharging, apis. mel. for hot, shiny red abscesses, merc. sol. for mouth abscesses, silicea to help a long-term abscess to heal.

Anal glands

The anal glands lie just below a dog's and cat's anus and act as the animal's scent glands. They usually empty every time your pet has a bowel movement. However, constipation or insufficient roughage in the diet can prevent this from happening and can lead to swollen, blocked and infected anal glands. Overweight or elderly animals can also be prone to anal gland problems. Signs of this in your pet are excessive licking of their bottom, itchy anus, dragging their bottom along the ground or crying out during bowel movements. If your pet is in a lot of pain or the condition does not improve within a few days, consult your vet, since the anal glands may need to be surgically drained.

Diet – This is the primary treatment. Give your pet a natural preservative-free diet with adequate roughage. Psyllium husks added to food add natural vegetable fibre to the diet and can help to ease the problem. You can also add raw, grated carrot to their food, or some chopped-up prunes or figs. Vegetable oil added to food also helps to lubricate the bowel. Raw garlic is an intestinal antiseptic and can be mixed in with their food or use garlic capsules if they don't like the taste. Provide plenty of fresh water (see Chapters 4 and 5).

Bach flower remedies – Use crab apple for cleansing.

Biochemical tissue salts – Use silica for repeated anal gland problems, as it encourages the discharge of pus.

Grapefruit-seed extract – Add 10 drops to an eggcup of water and wipe around the anal glands for a potent antibiotic. Grapefruit-seed extract can also be added to their food daily.

Herbs – Use aloe vera juice taken internally and add raw garlic to their food. Soak fenugreek seeds in warm water overnight, then mix the seeds into their food and give them the liquid to drink. Many animals love the taste of curry and enjoy fenugreek in their food. If using a brown-rice-based diet, cook the seeds in with their rice. Diluted witch hazel can be dabbed on the glands if they are particularly swollen.

Homoeopathy – Use hepar. sulph. for infected glands, silicea for repeated anal gland problems, arnica may also help with inflammation and discomfort.

Exercise – Exercise is also important to help eliminate toxins from the body and keep the anal glands emptying properly.

Coat problems

Coat problems include hair loss, dull coat, unhealthy-looking coat, dandruff and coarse or matted coat.

The condition of your pet's coat tells you a lot about their general health. A dull coat is one of the first signs of deteriorating health, whilst actual hair loss is a sign that the deterioration is more serious. Hair loss can be all over the body or in small, localised patches. Many factors can lead to hair loss or an unhealthy coat, including poor diet, parasites, hormonal problems, digestive problems, allergies, bacterial or fungal infections, weakened immune system, liver or kidney problems.

Diet – A good, healthy diet is the key to a healthy-looking coat. The first thing you need to do is change your pet's food to a natural, additive-free diet or allergy diet. Grated, raw carrot and beetroot help to cleanse the liver and kidneys. Add brewer's yeast regularly to their food for extra B vitamins (or yeast-free B-complex supplement if a yeast allergy is suspected). Oil of evening primrose or linseed oil, and fish-liver oil will help restore the coat's shine. Apple cider vinegar mixed into the food adds potassium to the diet. Also give zinc (5–20mg daily), vitamin C (500–5,000mg daily), green super-foods, plus a good-quality, multi-mineral and vitamin supplement for dogs or cats (see Chapters 4 and 5).

Aromatherapy – Rosemary is invigorating and may be massaged into dull coats or directly onto bald patches where there is hair loss. (Put a few drops in a base oil such as olive oil or sunflower oil.) Other useful oils include lavender, thyme, tea tree and pine. Your local pet shop may also stock a natural herbal shampoo, such as seaweed and birch, which relieves surface skin problems and deters fleas and parasites. Tea tree and rosemary are good for treating dandruff. New Seasons (UK) stock a wide range of aromatherapy products for pets (see Chapter 8).

Bach flower remedies – Use crab apple for general cleansing and detoxifying.

Biochemical tissue salts – Use kali. sulph., nat. mur., silica for hair loss, nat. mur. and kali. sulph. for dandruff.

Grapefruit-seed extract – Add 10 drops to an eggcup of oil or water and apply to the affected area twice a day.

Herbs – Use aloe vera, cat's claw, garlic, nettle, dandelion, seaweed. Aloe vera juice and raw garlic taken internally are very cleansing. Aloe vera spray can be used externally. Seaweed or kelp tablets help thyroid function and restore health to the coat. Nettles and dandelions cleanse the system and support the kidneys and liver. Cat's claw and garlic enhance the immune system. There are some excellent ready-made herbal skin treatments on the market; for example, Hilton Herbs (UK) make a skin and coat formula which includes apple cider vinegar, honey, clivers, nettle, kelp, garlic, burdock and calendula (see Chapter 13).

Homoeopathy – Use arsen. alb. for dandruff, or try sulphur. Use nat. mur. for hair loss, arsen. alb. for hair loss with itchiness, lycopodium for elderly and balding pets, pulsatilla for hair loss related to female hormone problems. If allergies are suspected, Ainsworths (UK) supplies a number of remedies to counteract specific allergies, such as pollen (see Chapter 14).

Grooming – Both cats and dogs will benefit from regular grooming to stimulate hair growth.

Eczema and dermatitis

(Also see Coat problems and Immune system.)

Symptoms include general itching and scratching, along with inflamed red sores on the skin which can become infected. In long-term, chronic cases the skin can become dry and scaly, or it may be greasy, and some of the animal's hair may fall out. There are many causes of eczema, including allergies, parasites, contact with chemicals, bacterial infections and autoimmune skin diseases.

Diet – Follow the dietary guidelines for allergic pets in Chapter 4. Chronic, long-term eczema responds well to fasting since it helps to cleanse the body of impurities. This can be on a one-day-a-week basis if the condition has been around for some time.

Add kelp and one of the green super-foods to the diet plus vitamin E (50–300iu daily), zinc (5–20mg daily), vitamin C (500–3,000mg daily), vitamin A (5,000–10,000iu daily), brewer's yeast or a yeast-free B complex daily, plus oils, such as evening primrose oil and fish oil or linseed oil daily (see Chapters 4 and 5).

Environment – Check your pet's environment for allergens, such as moulds, pollens, house dust, house-dust mites, fleas or anything that could be causing an allergic reaction. Keep their bed clean and aired.

Aromatherapy – Tea tree oil can be massaged into the skin. Put a few drops in a base oil like olive oil or sunflower and massage straight onto the affected area. Tea tree is antiseptic and soothing and helps to heal sore skin. Lavender is also soothing to the skin. Essential oils can be mixed into a base cream, such as olive oil cream, and used as an ointment on the skin. Some come ready-made as creams for external use.

Bach flower remedies – Crab apple is the cleansing remedy and helps to clear out toxins and bacterial infections. It also helps to rid the animal of unwanted emotions.

Biochemical tissue salts – Use combination D for minor skin complaints, kali. phos. for greasy, scaly skin, kali. sulph. for dry skin, silica for skin that is slow to heal.

Grapefruit-seed extract – Add 5–15 drops, 2 or 3 times daily to your pet's food to combat bacterial and fungal infections. This can also be diluted (add 10 drops to an eggcup of water) and used externally as an antiseptic wash.

Herbs – Use garlic, nettle, aloe vera, valerian, milk thistle. Liquid garlic can be used externally to heal and clean sore skin areas. Garlic taken internally has antiseptic and healing properties and helps to remove internal parasites and fight infection. You can use it raw in your pet's food or buy ready-made garlic tablets. Nettles are cleansing and purifying and can be used fresh or in tablet form. Aloe vera gel can be spread directly onto the skin and has a soothing and healing effect. Aloe vera is also available as a spray for use on animals. Valerian has a calming effect on the animal's nervous system. Milk thistle helps liver function; many skin conditions have their root in impaired liver function. Licorice has anti-inflammatory and immune-boosting properties. Hilton Herbs (UK) make a skin and coat formula which includes apple cider vinegar, honey, clivers, nettle, kelp, garlic, burdock and calendula (see Chapter 13).

Homoeopathy – Sulphur is the main remedy for skin ailments, especially with redness and warm, itchy skin. Use cantharis for burning, angry skin eruptions, hepar. sulph. for infected, discharging sores on the skin, graphites for eczema with discharge. Try thuja if you suspect vaccine damage.

Scratching

Scratching can be caused by a number of things, but the two most common triggers are allergies and parasites. A herbal shampoo, such as seaweed and birch, will help to relieve scratching. You could also bathe your pet in water with a few drops of tea tree added. The most important first step, though, is to change your pet's food to a natural allergy-free diet and filtered or bottled water. (Also see Eczema and dermatitis and Coat problems, in this section.)

Smelly animals

A smelly animal is a sure sign that the animal is toxic or is eating an inadequate diet. The smell comes through the skin since this is a major organ of elimination and when the smell is noticeable it means the body is labouring under a heavy toxic load. Usually poor diet, poor digestion and poor elimination are at the root of this. If your pet has constipation or diarrhoea these need to be addressed as well, along with changing to a natural additive-free diet. If bad breath is a problem, have their teeth and mouth checked out by your vet. Other causes of smelly animals are skin problems, worm infestations, and glandular disorders. (Also see Digestive Problems, Ear Problems, Parasites, Skin and coat in Chapter 17.)

Diet – A change to a natural additive-free regime may be enough to sort the problem out. Many animals will benefit from an occasional day's fast to help them eliminate toxins from the body. Use probiotics and digestive enzymes, plus a good-quality, multi-mineral and vitamin supplement for dogs or cats (see Chapters 4 and 5).

Bach flower remedies – Use crab apple for cleansing.

Herbs – Aloe vera and garlic are great internal cleansers. Dandelion and nettle help to detox the liver and kidneys.

Homoeopathy – Use nux vomica, given in acute or chronic doses depending on the condition.

Bathing – Both dogs and cats can benefit from being washed. Some cats do not clean themselves properly which may be the cause of their odour. Pets can be bathed in water with lemon juice or tea tree oil added or use a natural herbal shampoo.

Exercise – Exercise is also important to help eliminate toxins from the body.

Warts

Warts grow on the skin and are usually harmless. They can grow singly or come in clusters and often come and go naturally on younger animals who have strong immune systems. Older or weak animals may not naturally get rid of their warts. If a wart gets damaged it can bleed or become infected. It is thought that warts are caused by a virus, and may appear after vaccination.

Diet – Change to a natural preservative-free diet to keep the immune system strong and to lessen the toxic load in the body. Garlic is a great internal cleanser and immune booster and can be added raw to food. Use a good-quality, multi-mineral and vitamin supplement for cats or dogs. Make sure it contains zinc, vitamin C, vitamin A and all the B vitamins. Vitamin E capsules can be opened and dabbed directly onto warts (see Chapters 4 and 5).

Aromatherapy – Tea tree or lemon oil can be dabbed directly onto warts.

Bach flower remedies – Use crab apple for cleansing. Another useful flower remedy for warts is pansy which is one of the FES and California Research Essences.

Biochemical tissue salts – Use kali. mur. and nat. mur. given together.

Grapefruit-seed extract – Use 1 drop directly on the wart twice daily.

Herbs – Use echinacea or cat's claw taken internally to boost the immune system, aloe vera taken internally as a general cleanser. Tree of life can be used topically for treating warts.

Homoeopathy – Thuja is the main remedy for warty growths. You can also dab thuja tincture onto the wart on a daily basis.

SPAYING AND NEUTERING

Whether to spay female pets or neuter male pets comes down to personal choice. However, many unwanted kittens and puppies can be prevented if animals that are free to roam are spayed or neutered. Neutered cats are less likely to roam or spray in the house and dogs often become gentler, less aggressive pets. This does require surgery, but there is a lot you can do afterwards to help with the healing process (see Operations). It is a debatable point whether either operation causes long-term health problems; you have to make what you feel is the right decision for you and your pet.

Although the operation can be costly, the PDSA (UK) helps those on low incomes by providing free health care for their pets. The best time to have an animal spayed or neutered is once your pet has reached sexual maturity, assuming you are not going to breed from them. I would recommend that you wait for at least one or two seasons in a female before having them spayed.

Diet – A preservative-free diet and supplement regime will help to speed their recovery from the operation. Your pet may also benefit from a short, liquid fast immediately after surgery to give its body a chance to heal. Useful additions to the diet to aid recovery include plenty of good-quality protein, raw vegetables, garlic, vitamins A, C and E, B complex, zinc, calcium and magnesium. (See Chapters 4 and 5 for advice on diet and supplements.) Vitamin E capsules can be opened and the contents rubbed onto operation scars to assist the healing process.

Bach flower remedies – Rescue remedy will help to calm an animal before and after their operation. Clematis helps them to recover from the anaesthetic. Use crab apple for cleansing after an anaesthetic, olive for an exhausted animal.

Grapefruit-seed extract – 5–15 drops added to food, 2 or 3 times daily as an antibiotic. It can also be used externally as a wash to keep the operation wound free of infection.

Herbs – Comfrey can be taken internally or used externally to promote rapid healing. Comfrey cream can be applied topically on the operation wound. Echinacea or cat's claw taken internally helps to boost the immune system.

Homoeopathy – Use aconite immediately before and afterwards for stress and fear, arnica for bruising, hypericum helps to relieve pain and repair damaged tissue.

General resources

Newsletters and journals
UK
Canine Health Concern
(Quarterly newsletter)
See Chapter 4 for details.

The Homoeopathic Society For Animal Welfare (Quarterly newsletter.)
Newparc, Llanrhidian, Gower, Swansea SA3 1HA
Tel/Fax: 01792 390943

Canada
Canine Health Naturally
('The thinking person's complementary care for canines.')
Tel: (604) 921 7784

US
Love of Animals
(Natural care and healing monthly newsletter for dogs and cats.)
Tel: (800) 711 2292

Holistic vets/Practitioners
UK
See relevant chapters for contacts.

US
The American Holistic Veterinary Medical Association
2214 Old Emmorton Road, Bel Air, MD 21015
Tel: (410) 569 0795
Fax: (410) 569 2346
Email: ahvma@compuserve.com
Internet: www.altvetmed.com
(Excellent source of information concerning animal health. Referrals to holistic veterinarians. Call or write, sending a sae, for a list of vets who are members in your local area.)

Australia
Holistic Animal Therapy Association of Australia
PO Box 202, Ormond, Victoria, 3204
Tel/Fax: (03) 9578 3710

Food supplements
See Chapter 5 for details.

Natural remedies
See relevant chapters for details.

Bibliography

Allport, Richard, BVetMed, VetMFHom, MRCVS, *Heal your Cat the Natural Way*; Mitchell Beazley, 1997.

Allport, Richard, BVetMed, VetMFHom, MRCVS, *Heal your Dog the Natural Way*; Mitchell Beazley, 1997.

Bradford, Nikki, *The Hamlyn Encyclopaedia of Complementary Health*; Hamlyn, 1996.

Burton Goldberg Group, The, *Alternative Medicine, the Definitive Guide*; Future Medicine Publishing, Inc., 1993.

Day, Christopher, MA VetMB, MRCVS, VetFFHom, *Homoeopathy, First Aid for Pets;* Chinham Publications, 1992.

Drury, Susan, *Tea Tree Oil, a Medicine Kit in a Bottle*; The C.W. Daniel Company Ltd, 1991.

Earle, Liz, *Liz Earle's Quick Guides – Aromatherapy*; Boxtree Ltd, 1994.

Frazier, Anitra, with Norma Eckroate, *The New Natural Cat*; Plume, 1990.

Harper, Joan, *The Healthy Cat and Dog Cook Book*; Pet Press, 1975.

Harvey, Clare G and Amanda Cochrane, *The Encyclopaedia of Flower Remedies*; Thorsons, 1995.

Goldstein, Martin, DVM, *The Nature of Animal Healing*; Random House, 1999.

Grosjean, Nelly, *Veterinary Aromatherapy*; The C.W. Daniel Company Limited, 1994.

Hoffman, David, *The New Holistic Herbal*; Element Books, 1990.

Hunter, Francis MRCVS, VetMFHom, *Homoeopathic First Aid Treatment for Pets*; Thorsons, 1988.

Lararus, Pat, *Keep your Pet Healthy the Natural Way*; Keats Publishing, Inc., 1986.

McKay, Pat, *Reigning Cats and Dogs*; Oscar Publications, 1992.

MacLeod, George, *Homoeopathy for Pets*; Wigmore Publications Ltd, 1981.

O'Driscoll, Catherine, *What Vets Don't Tell you about Vaccines*; Abbeywood Publishing (Vaccines) Ltd, 1997.

Pitcairn, Richard, DVM, PhD, and Susan Hubble Pitcairn, *Dr Pitcairn's Complete Guide to Natural Health for Dogs and Cats*; Rodale Books, 1995.

Raymonde-Hawkins MBE, M and George MacLeod, *The Raystede Handbook of Homoeopathic Remedies for Animals*; The C.W. Daniel Company Ltd, 1985.

Stanway, Andrew, Dr, *A Guide to Biochemical Tissue Salts*; Van Dyke Books, 1982.

Stein, Diane, *The Natural Remedy Book for Dogs And Cats*; The Crossing Press, 1994.

Stein, Diane, *Natural Healing for Dogs and Cats*; The Crossing Press, 1993.

Vlamis, Gregory, *Rescue Remedy, The Healing Power of Bach Flower Rescue Remedy*; Thorsons, 1990.

At-a-glance guide to Bach Flower Remedies

Fear

Terror	Rock Rose
Fear of known things	Mimulus
Fear of mind giving way	Cherry Plum
Fears and worries of unknown origin	Aspen
Fear or over-concern for others	Red Chestnut

Over-care for the welfare of others

Selfishly possessive	Chicory
Over-enthusiasm	Vervain
Domineering, inflexible	Vine
Intolerance	Beech
Self-repression, self-denial	Rock Water

Over-sensitivity to influences and ideas

Mental torment behind a brave face	Agrimony
Weak-willed and subservient	Centaury
Protection from change and outside influences	Walnut
Hatred, envy, jealousy	Holly

Loneliness

Proud, aloof	Water Violet
Impatience	Impatiens
Self-centredness, self-concern	Heather

Despondency or despair

Lack of confidence	Larch
Self-reproach, guilt	Pine
Overwhelmed by responsibility	Elm
Extreme mental anguish	Sweet Chestnut
After-effects of shock	Star of Bethlehem
Resentment	Willow
Exhausted but struggles on	Oak
Self-hatred, sense of uncleanliness	Crab Apple

Uncertainty

Seeks advice and confirmation from others	Cerato
Indecision	Scleranthus
Discouragement, despondency	Gentian
Hopelessness and despair	Gorse
'Monday morning' feeling	Hornbeam
Uncertainty as to the correct path in life	Wild Oat

Insufficient interest in present circumstances

Dreaminess, lack of interest in present	Clematis
Lives in past	Honeysuckle
Resignation, apathy	Wild Rose
Lack of energy	Olive
Unwanted mental arguments	White Chestnut
Deep gloom with no origin	Mustard
Failure to learn from past mistakes	Chestnut Bud

Index

Entries in **bold** refer to tables

A

abscesses 208–9
accidents 74, 97, 139, 144, 189, 190
acid/alkaline balance 13, 35, 156
    see also pH
aconite 119, 122, 126, 140, 189, 190
acupuncture 45–53
    conditions helped by 49
    and length of treatment 51
    as preventive medicine 49
acupuncture points 48
ageing 22, 23, 24
aggression 149–50
AIDS 41
alkalinity *see* acid/alkaline balance
allergens 12, 14, 212
allergies 159–60, 180
    in food 16, 19, 23–4, 34
aloe vera 33, 140
    in first aid kit 111, 137
aloofness 83, 87
anaemia 31, 158–9
anal glands 209–10
anger 86
anorexia 161
antibiotics 138
antioxidants 13–14
antiseptic 139

anxiety 62, 152–3
    and flower essences 81, 83
appetite 160–2
    problems 50, 161–2
apple cider vinegar 33
Arnica 126, 137, 140
aromatherapy 54–64
    and abscesses 208
    and aggression 150
    and coat problems 210
    and colds 207
    conditions helped by 58
    and coughs 205–6
    and fleas 196
    and grief 151
    and infectious diseases 181
    length of treatment 60
    and operations 193
    and other treatments 61
    safety of 59
    and sprains 192
    and spraying 154
    and ticks 198
arthritis 186–8
    and acupuncture 49, 51
    and essential oils 58, 61
    and herbal medicine 104, 107, 109
    and hip dysplasia 190
    and spinal problems 191
    and steroids 48

Arthur, Richard 72
aspen 86, 88
asthma 180, 194, 204
astragalus 111
autism 41

B
Bach, Edward (Dr) 78, 80
Bach flower remedies **220**
    see also flower essences
bacteria 16, 36
basset-hounds 73, 191
bathing 6, 57, 197, 213
bed and bedding 5–6, 196
beech 88
behavioural problems 2, 94, **148**,
    149
belladonna 126
bereavement 151
    see also death
biochemical tissue salts
    see tissue salts
birth and labour 203
biting 149–50
bladder and bladder stones 182–3
bleeding 139–40
blood 29, 156, 157–9
    and iron 31
    and ticks 197–8
    in urine 182
blood pressure 32, 185
blood sugar levels 165, 166, 170
bone-meal 34
bones 16, 29
    and diet 30, 31
    fractured 137–8, 189
    and magnesium 32
    and vitamins 30
bossiness 89
boundaries 5
breath 162, 213
brewer's yeast 34
bronchitis 205
bruising 57, 140
burns and scalds 137, 140–1

C
calcium 31, 34
calcium fluoride 67
calcium phosphate 65, 67
calcium sulphate 67
calendula 126, 137
cancer 4, **148**, 155–6, 180
    and flea treatments 194
    and vitamins 30–1
car sickness 58, 87
carbohydrates 18–19
cardiovascular system **148**, 156–9
cartilage 35, 187
Casley, Christy 98
cataracts 178
cat's claw 111
catteries 43, 57, 61
charcoal 136
chestnut bud 86
'chi' 46, 92
chicory 86, 88
'Chinese diagnosis' 47–8
Chinese medicine see acupuncture
chiropractic 70–6
    conditions treated 73
    means of action 71–2
    and musculo-skeletal problems 187
    safety of 74
cholesterol 36
circulatory system 156, 157–8
Clark, Hulda (Dr) 199–200
clematis 86, 88
coat and coat problems **148**, 207–14,
    210
colds 206–7
colic 162–3
colitis 163–4
collies 95
comfrey 111
compresses 57
conjunctivitis 178–9
consciousness 143, 144
constipation 164–5, 209
    and elderly pets 24
    and fruit 20

and psyllium 37, 103, 209
and smelly animals 213
'convenience food for pets' 10
coughs 205–6
cuts and grazes 141
   see also wounds
cystitis 13, 183–4

D
dachshunds 73, 191
dairy produce 16–17
dandruff 210
death 62, 86–7, 151
   and acupuncture 49
   and flower essences 85
   and healing 94, 96
degenerative diseases 42
depression 151
dermatitis 211–12
detoxification 33
   see also toxins
diabetes 4, 165–6
diagnosis and chiropractic 72
diarrhoea 30, 166–8
diet 3, 9–27
   and abscesses 208
   and aggression 150
   and anaemia 158–9
   and anal glands 209
   and anxiety 152–3
   and appetite problems 161, 162
   and arthritis 186–7, 187, 187–8
   and broken bones 189
   and cancer 155–6
   change of 21
   and coat problems 210
   and colds 206–7
   and colic 162
   and colitis 163
   and constipation 164
   core of a healthy life 3–4
   and cystitis 183–4
   and dental problems 172
   and diabetes 166
   and diarrhoea 167

and ear problems 177
and eczema 211
and eye problems 178, 179
and false pregnancy 201
and fleas 196
and food allergies 160
and fur balls 169
and grief 151
healthy 10–11
and heart conditions 157
and hip dysplasia 190
and hyperactivity 152
and illness prevention 146, 147
and incontinence 184–5
and infectious diseases 181
and infertility 202
and joint dislocation 190–1
and kidney disease 182–3,
   185–6
and liver disease 169–70
and milk production 201
necessity for 5
optimum 14–15
and overweight animals 174–5
and pregnancy 188, 190, 200,
   203–4
and skin and coat conditions
   207
and smelly animals 213
and spaying 215
and sprains 192
and stomach problems 171
and stress 154
and vomiting 173–4
and warts 214
and weight loss 175–6
and worms 199
   see also individual items
      eg protein
diffusers 57
digestive enzymes 170
digestive problems 36, **148**, 159–76
   and grapefruit-seed extract 35
   and peppermint 62
   and tinned food 13

▼

discipline 5
diseases, infectious 180–2
drowsiness 86
drugs 1, 2

E
ear mites 194, 195
ear problems **148**, 176–7
echinacea 111–12
eczema 211–12
elderly pets 22, 23, 24
electrolyte balance 32, 33
   see also acid/alkaline balance; pH
energy 92–3
   channels 46
   of essential oils 55
   and flower essences 79
   in food 22–3
   and healing 91–3
   and homoeopathy 118
environment 78, 196, 212
enzymes 12, 19
   digestive 34
epilepsy 59
essential oils 54, 55–8
   healing properties 55–6
   purchase of 63
   usage 56–9
eucalyptus 61
evening primrose oil 34
exercise
   and arthritis 188
   and behaviour 149
   and constipation 164
   and diabetes 166
   and heart disease 157
   and joint problems 186
   necessity for 5
   and overweight animals 175
   and smelly animals 213
   and spinal disease 191, 192
exhaustion 87
eyebright 112
eyes and eye problems 29, **148**,
   178–80

F
faeces 198
false pregnancy 201
fasting
   and allergies 23, 171
   and arthritis 187
   and change in diet 21
   and diarrhoea 167
   and eczema 211
   and healing 26–7
   and honey 36
   and operations 193
   and skin and coat conditions
      207
   and smelly animals 213
   and stomach problems 171
   and vomiting 173–4
fatigue 88
fats and oils 17–18
fatty acids 17, 18, 34
fear 87, 88, 152–3
feline urology syndrome 184
fibre
   from carbohydrates 18
   and constipation 164, 209
   and elderly pets 24
   in fruit and vegetables 19, 20
   and worms 199
first-aid
   and aromatherapy 59
   and herbal medicine 107, 109
   and natural remedies 136–45
fish and fish oil 16, 18
fish oil 34
Fisher, Sarah 56, 59, 61, 133
flatulence 168
flea collars 58
fleas and flea bites 113–14, 194,
   195–7, 198
   and essential oils 57, 61–2
   and herbal medicine 113–14
flower essences 77–90
   and aggression 150
   choice of 82–3
   and common problems 80–1

and death 85
dosage 84
effectiveness 79
and infectious diseases 181
and operations 194
and pregnancy 204
as preventive medicine 85
storage of 85
and travel sickness 173
and weight loss 176
flower remedy medicine chest
    86–9
fluid balance 32, 185
food 13, 14, 20, 22, 88
    allergies 24, 159–60, 171
    commercially prepared 12
    supplements 28–40
    see also diet
food allergens see allergens
France 58
frankincense 60, 61
fresh air 5
fruit 20
fur balls 164, 168–9

G
garlic 34–5, 112, 197
gelsemium 126
geranium 61
germ theory of disease 43
German shepherd dogs 189, 191
ginger 112
glucosamine sulphate 35
Goldstein, Martin 41, 42
Gould, Helen 50, 52
Govan, Alasdair MacFarlane 46–7, 49,
    50–1
grains 18–19
grapefruit-seed extract 35–6
    and abscesses 208
    and anal glands 209
    and eczema 212
    and first-aid kit 138
    and infectious diseases 181
    and operations 194

and worms 199
gravel 182–3
green super-foods 35
greyhounds 73, 74
grief 87, 88, 151
grooming 6, 164, 211
    and fleas 196, 197
    and fur balls 168, 169
growth 32
gum disease 162
gums 29, 171–2

H
Hahnemann, Samuel 118
Harvey, Clare 79, 81, 85
healing 91–100
    action 93
    choice of 94
    conditions helped by 93–4
    distant 97
    and first-aid 97
    length of treatment 96
    and other therapies 97
heart and heart disease 4, 32, 156,
    157–8
hepar. sulph. 126
herbal medicine 101–16
    conditions aided 104–5
    dosage 110
    healing action 105–6
    and length of treatment 109
    means of action 102–3
    and other treatments 113
    preparation and dosage 108–10
    preventative action 106–7
    response to treatment 110–11
    side effects of 103–4
herbs 21
    and abscesses 208–9
    and anal glands 209
    and arthritis 188
    and broken bones 189
    and coat problems 211
    and constipation 165
    and coughs 206

and dental problems 172
and diarrhoea 168
in diet 112–13
and ear problems 177
and eczema 212
and eye problems 178, 179
and fleas 196–7
and food allergies 160
healing properties of 104
and infectious diseases 181–2
and infertility 202
and kidney disease 186
and liver disease 170
and mastitis 203
and operations 194
and overweight animals 175
and pregnancy 204
and spaying 215
and spinal problems 192
and sprains 192–3
and stomach problems 171
and travel sickness 173
and vomiting 174
and weight loss 176
hip dysplasia 189–90
holistic healing defined 2, 3
holly 86
homoeopathy 117–29, 174
    and abscesses 209
    advantages of 122–3
    alternative to vaccination 43–4
    and arthritis 188
    and broken bones 189
    and coat problems 211
    and colds 207
    conditions helped by 121–2
    and coughs 206
    and dental problems 172
    and diagnosis 119–20
    dosage 124–5
    and ear problems 177
    and eczema 212
    and energy or vibration 118
    and eye problems 178, 179
    and food allergies 160

    and healing reactions 120
    home use of 123
    and incontinence 185
    and kidney disease 186
    and mastitis 203
    and operations 194
    potency 120–1, 123
    and pregnancy 204
    safety of 121
    and spinal problems 192
    and travel sickness 173
honey 36
honeysuckle 86–7, 88
hormonal problems 50, 201
hornbeam 88
horse dung 102
human-animal bond 78, 131, 132
hyperactivity 87, 152
hypericum 126, 138

I
immune system 3, **148**, 180–2
    and arthritis 187
    and cancer 155
    and diet 25
    and essential oils 56
    and grapefruit-seed extract 35
    and honey 36
    and mange 197
    and operations 193
    and parasites 194
    and probiotics 36
    and vitamin C 30
    and worming 199
    and zinc 32
immunisation programs 41
incontinence 184–5
infections 180–2
infertility 202
inflammation 138, 139
inhalation of essential oils 57
insect bites and stings 142
insulin 165
intelligence 131
iodine 36

iron 31–2
iron phosphate 67

J
joint problems **148**, 186, 190–1
  see also musculo-skeletal
    problems

K
kelp 36
kennel cough 180, 204, 205
kennels 43, 57, 61
  and vaccination 43
kidney conditions **148**, 182–6
  and dried food 13
  stones 182–3
  and tinned food 13
kittens 22, 25
  and calcium 31
  and vaccinations 42

L
labradors 95, 119, 189
lactation 31
larch 88
lavender 61–2, 138
lead 13
lecithin 36
leftovers 21
lice 194, 197
life force 46, 92–3
  and essential oils 55
  and food 20
  see also energy
liver conditions 169–70
  and acupuncture 50
  and homoeopathy 122
  and tinned food 13
loneliness 86–7
Lonsdale, Tom 11

M
MacFarlane Govan, Alasdair
    see Govan, Alasdair MacFarlane
MacLeod, George 119

McTimoney, John 71
McTimoney chiropractic method 71,
    73
magnesium 32
magnesium phosphate 67
  and muscles 65
  and nerves 65
mange 197
manipulation techniques 71–2
marjoram 62
massage 57–8
  see also T-touch massage
mastitis 201, 202–3
meals 22
meat 15–16
melissa 62
mercury 13, 21, 126–7
meridians 46
milk production 201, 202, 203
milk thistle 112
mimulus 87, 88
mineral salts *see* tissue salts
minerals 29, 31–3
  in food 17–18
Moshe, Dr 131
multi-vitamins 31, 32–3
muscle 32, 62
musculo-skeletal problems 73, **148**,
    186–93
  and acupuncture 49
  and chiropractic 70, 71
  and glucosamine sulphate 35

N
nerves and nervous system 29, 32,
    72
  and acupuncture 50
  and flea treatments 194
  and herbs 62, 103
nervousness 86, 152–3
neutering **148**, 214–15
Newman, Christine 82
nosodes 43
nutrition *see* diet
nux vomica 127

O

obese animals 174–5
offal 16
olive 87
operations **148**, 193–4
osteoporosis 189
overheating 144
overweight animals 174–5, 187

P

pain and pain relief 35, 138, **148**
    and acupuncture 49, 51
    and magnesium 32
pancreas 165, 170
paralysis 191–2
parasites **148**, 194–200
    cure for 199–200
    and essential oils 57
    and garlic 34
Pasteur, Louis 43, 180
PDSA 215
peppermint 62
pesticides 2
pet food see food
pH balance 32, 33, 35, 36
    see also acid/alkaline balance
pining 151
plant essential oils see essential
    oils
play 6
poisoning 142–3
    see also toxins
police dogs 74
pollution 2, 155, 159
possessiveness 86, 88
potassium 32, 33
potassium chloride 67
potassium phosphate 67
potassium sulphate 67
'prana' 92
pregnancy 31, 33, **148**, 200–4
    and diet 188, 203–4
preventative medicine 4, 147
probiotics 36–7, 164
protein 15–17, 17

and elderly pets 24
    metabolism 182
    substandard 13
psyllium husks 37, 112
puppies
    and diet 22, 25, 31, 190
    and vaccinations 42

R

reproductive system 31, 32, 50
rescue remedy 80, 82, 83, 86
    and accidents 139, 189
    in first aid kit 87, 89, 137
resentment 83
respiratory diseases **148**, 204–5
retrievers 189
rheumatism 186–8
    and essential oils 58, 61
    and hip dysplasia 189
Rhus tox 127
Rohrbach, John 2, 102–3, 105,
    114
roughage see fibre
roundworms see worms
routine 6

S

Saxton, J.G.C. 82
Schuessler, Wilhelm (Dr) 65
scleranthus 87
scratching 213
self-confidence 88
self-healing and plant oils 55
sensitivity 91–2
setters 119, 176
shock 143
    and aconite 140, 190–1
    and arnica 137
    and flower essences 83, 84
sickness 167
    and eating 26
    and fur balls 168–9
    and poisoning 142
    and stomach problems 170
    see also vomiting

side effects of drugs 2
silicon dioxide 68
skeletal system 70
skin and skin conditions 29, **148**,
    180, 207–14
  and essential oils 61
  and homoeopathy 122
  and tea tree 62–3
slipped disc 191
slippery elm 112
smelly animals 213
smoking 205
socialising 6, 89
sodium 32
sodium chloride 67
sodium phosphate 68
sodium sulphate 68
spaniels 176
spaying **148**, 214–15
spine and spinal disease 191–2
  and acupuncture 49, 50–1
  and chiropractic 71
spondylitis and spondylosis 191
sporting dogs 74
sprains and strains 192–3
spraying 154
star of Bethlehem 87, 88–9
steroid drugs 48
stomach problems 170–1
stress 3, 62, 154
  and human-animal bond 79
  on immune system 180
  and milk production 201
sugar 14
sulphur 127
sunshine 5
sunstroke 144
swimming 6
  see also bathing; exercise

T
T-touch massage 130–5
  conditions treated 132
  definition 130–1
  effectiveness 131–2

length of treatment 134
  means of practice 134
tapeworms see worms
tea tree 62–3, 138
teeth 16, 29, 171–2
  and bones 25
  and diet 30, 31
  and magnesium 32
  and smelly animals 213
  and vitamins 30
Tellington-Jones, Linda 130, 131
Third-Carter, June 119–20, 122, 123,
    127
thyme 56
thymol 56
thyroid 36
ticks 197–8
tissue salts 65–9
  administration and dosage 66–7,
    68
  and colds 207
  conditions helped by 66
  healing mechanism of 66
  and other treatments 69
  specificity 66
  storage 69
toxins 26
  and arthritis 187
  and cancer 155
  and charcoal 136
  in commercial pet food 12–13
  and diarrhoea 167
  and fasting 23
  and kidney disease 185
  and liver function 169
  and psyllium 37
  and skin conditions 207
  and smelly animals 213
  see also poisoning
training of dogs 86
trauma 87, 88–9, 143
travel sickness 172–3
  see also sickness
treats 20, 25–6
tuna fish 13, 21

U
underweight animals 175–6
urinary problems **148**, 154, 165, 182–6, 183

V
vaccinations 2–3, 41, 41–4
    and behavioural problems 42
    and diet 23
    and warts 214
vegetables 19
vervain 87
vets 98, 105, 120, 146
vine 89
vitamins 12, 19, 29–31
    in food 17–18
    in fruit 20
    and kelp 36
    multi-vitamins 31, 33
    vitamin A 29
    vitamin B 29, 34, 36
    vitamin D 30
    vitamin E 30–1, 37, 145
Vlamis, Gregory: *Rescue Remedy* 82, 85
vomit and vomiting 173–4, 198

see also sickness

W
walnut 89
warts 214
water 22
water violet 87, 89
weight and weight problems 22, 174–6
wheat-germ oil 37
witch hazel 112, 139
work for dogs 6, 73
worms 194, 195, 198–9
    and diet 25
    and garlic 34
wounds 144–5
    and calendula 137
    and herbal medicine 107
    and vitamin C 30
    and zinc 32

Y
yin and yang 47

Z
zinc 32